SHIP MOMS

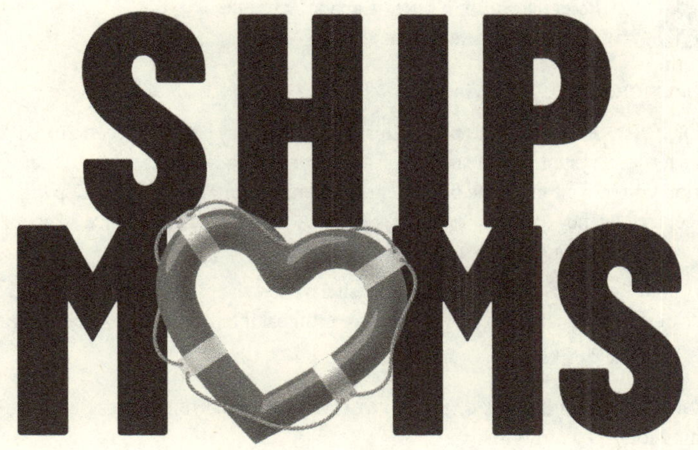

SHIP MOMS

TRUE TALES OF LOVE AND LUST AT SEA

JEN WINSOR

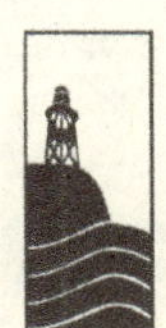

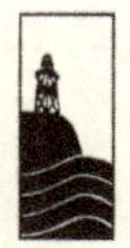

BREAKWATER
P.O. Box 2188, St. John's, NL Canada A1C 6E6
WWW.BREAKWATERBOOKS.COM

LIBRARY AND ARCHIVES CANADA CATALOGUING IN PUBLICATION
Ship Moms / by Jen Winsor.
Winsor, Jen, author
Canadiana (print) 20250166488 | Canadiana (ebook) 20250166496
ISBN 9781778530616 (softcover) | isbn 9781778530623 (EPUB)
LCSH: Cruise ships—Employees—Biography. |

PAGE LAYOUT: Nadine Hodder

THE PUBLISHER GRATEFULLY ACKNOWLEDGES THE SUPPORT OF
The Canada Council for the Arts
The Government of Canada through the Department of Heritage, and
The Government of Newfoundland and Labrador through the Department of Tourism, Culture, Arts and Recreation

Canada Council for the Arts Conseil des arts du Canada

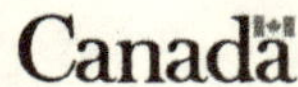

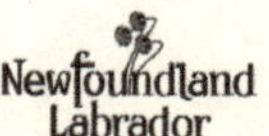

PRINTED AND BOUND IN CANADA.

Breakwater Books is committed to choosing papers and materials for our books that help to protect our environment. To this end, this book is made of FSC®-certified and other controlled material.

This book by, about, and for women, is dedicated to two men. Go figure.

For Gabriel and Luiz, who made me a ship mom.

I love you both so friggin' much.

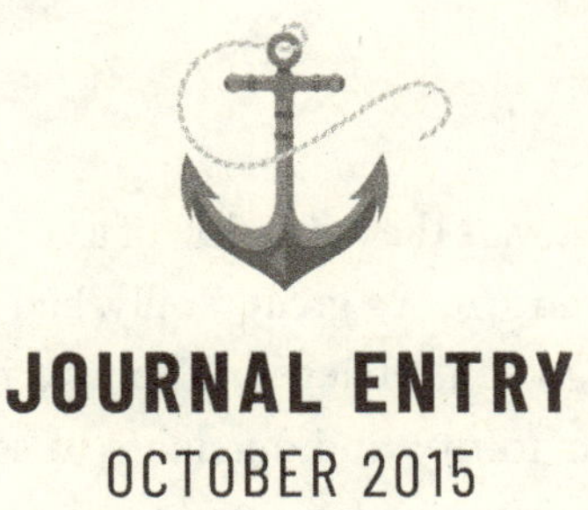

JOURNAL ENTRY

OCTOBER 2015

On the flight from Newfoundland to Port Canaveral, Florida, I cried as we took off. The man next to me gave me a tissue and said, "Something very special about this place." He'd assumed correctly what my tears were about, and I nodded in agreement. I'm equally excited and terrified about this new adventure. It's hard to leave Newfoundland. My safe little rock. The comfort of family and friends. But perhaps I am going for perspective. Going to learn about myself and the world. To find things bigger than myself. To seek the great.

What do I want from life anyway?

Obviously, it's not the career, husband, and house. I had all that and let it go. I wanted more. If my body isn't going to make a baby, then what's Plan B for my life? Travel. Experience. This is the hardest thing I have ever done, to walk away, but I'm doing it for us. For me and for him. A better life for us both, where we can both be happy. I'm sure he'll find a kind, beautiful woman who will want the same things.

Someday I will see him online with his beautiful family. I hope I feel joy for him and not regret . . . .

My partner, Robert, was the definition of a good guy. He was tall and handsome, came from a great family, had a well-paying job and an adorable golden retriever. When we met, I was struck by his kindness, maturity, and openness to settling down. We had a good relationship and seemed to want the same things in life.

I was working in the music industry at MusicNL, promoting music in my home province through programs, services, and events. It was my dream job. I loved the fun, fast-paced, and artistic environment. For any Newfoundland and Labrador music fans, my "era" was working with the legendary blues man, the late Denis Parker. My first conference with the association was the first showcase of Hey Rosetta!—undoubtedly one of the finest bands to ever emerge from the east coast of Canada. Some other fan favourites during my time there were the Once, Amelia Curran, Fortunate Ones, Chris Kirby and the Marquee, Mark Bragg, the Ennis Sisters, Mick Davis, Kellie Loder . . . the list could go on and on. Everywhere we travelled, MusicNL showcases—which featured our artists—had lineups around the block.

Being in a venue far away from home and hearing Shanneyganock bellow "Any Newfoundlanders in here tonight?"—*tonight* was, of course, pronounced *danite*—and watching a room full of partying people not from Newfoundland going nuts was always the best. As a huge music fan and hidden artist, it was hard not to adore being around the magic of supporting and presenting live music. And, of course, the partying.

Sometimes, too much partying.

All my life, I had an issue with knowing when to stop drinking once I started. Growing up in the Goulds, Newfoundland, I spent my teenage years beating the streets, scraping up enough money to eat fish and chips at Keith's and drink beer in the woods with my friends. In grade eight, while drinking London Dock stolen from someone's parents, I peed my pants in front of dozens of other kids. I don't remember how I got home, but later that night, my parents saved me from choking on my own vomit. Then they made me do alcohol-abuse counselling and grounded me for months.

Working in music was made more complicated by my love of alcohol because it was readily available everywhere and drinking was highly encouraged.

When we started dating, Robert, a former touring musician turned safety professional, loved how passionate I was about my work. But eventually, he grew annoyed by the job. He began to accuse me of looking for someone else, particularly someone in the music industry "with a beard." In his defence, I can admit now that it couldn't have been easy watching me gallivant all over Canada with bands, partying all night. I frequently drank too much, which compounded things.

A few years into the relationship, while blackout drunk, I cheated on Robert with a friend's roommate—an asshole, serial womanizer, and musician. Weeks later, riddled with guilt, I told Robert what had happened and begged him not to leave me.

He decided to stay and try to work it out, but things were never the same between us.

So how does a couple come back from this? Why, they get married and have babies, of course!

I'm sure Robert thought a baby would calm me down. And I think I did, too. We got hitched at a destination wedding in Jamaica, surrounded by friends and family. We started actively trying to have kids right away. But then months and months passed without even needing a pregnancy test. I would think back to when I was a teenager and frequented doctors with my mother about my messed-up periods. Maybe I should have fought more for answers instead of throwing birth control pills at the problem.

Everyone knew Robert and I were actively trying, and it added an extra layer of stress and pressure. It got to the point that our friends would hesitate to tell us when they got pregnant out of concern that it would hurt me.

I would always say, "Don't be silly. I am so happy for you!" Then, when I was alone, I'd bawl my eyes out. Of course I was happy for them, but it was stressful, and it took a toll on me. It started taking a toll on my relationship with Robert, too.

After a year of trying unsuccessfully to conceive, I was finally able to see a fertility specialist. It seemed I had irregular ovulation, which could be caused by a host of issues, but I had no other symptoms.

So what was the problem? The doctor couldn't say for sure. "It could likely be severe stress," she told me one day. "It can disrupt the body's normal function and lead to anovulation."

This got me questioning my life and what I wanted. I was happy, right? I loved my job and was living in a lovely home in the suburbs across the street from my childhood elementary school with a great, solid partner. I had nothing to complain about. So why was I questioning this perfect life?

As time passed with no pregnancy, no baby, I found myself filled with a feeling of dread and not understanding it. I felt cooped up in my house with my husband constantly out in the backyard shed, his man cave, insisting that was how he liked to relax. Was this the life I'd signed up for? How could I live in this perfect-for-children life we'd created and not have children?

The fact was, I couldn't.

I've always been terrible at confronting things, and this was especially true at that time in my life. I had no backbone and avoided conflict instead of having hard conversations. This had long-term effects and led to unresolved issues.

The truth, I realized, was that Robert and I were broken and not meant to be fixed.

Barely a year into our marriage, we separated. Robert took the separation as well as he could. Our divorce never needed mediators or anything of the sort, and there were no children, of course, which made things easier. The split was hard, but it was for the best for both of us.

I saw the fertility specialist at a couple more appointments before I was busted—no longer in a relationship. I was, therefore, "not actively trying" to get pregnant.

I moved into a downtown St. John's apartment a few blocks from my office and started to move on with my life. I still loved working in music, but the constant time spent in party spaces sponsored by alcohol companies was complex. Luckily for me, "harder drugs" mostly all had adverse effects on me. While cocaine typically makes people feel euphoric and boosts confidence, I would get paranoid, awkward, and quiet. Booze, on the other hand, made me happy, sociable, warm, and fuzzy. And it let me keep up with anyone who wanted to party, sing songs, listen to music, laugh a lot, and have deep conversations. For the most part, I was lucky to be surrounded by people who made sure I was okay.

There was, however, one incident right after my separation. One morning, a MusicNL board member found me asleep in a hospitality suite, still wearing my dress and dirty boots from the previous night. This likely contributed to why I was declined for a promotion not long after and couldn't move up in the organization. I remember Googling "Do I have a drinking problem?" around that time.

The fact is, if you are Googling that question, you likely do.

While generally happy, I still felt that longing to escape. Close friends remember my frequent singing of the Queen song "I Want to Break Free," an anthem for my overwhelming urge to get far away from everything I knew. But because I worked in the arts, I had no money.

So I started researching cruise ships in a desperate attempt to get as far away from Newfoundland as possible. My friend and a former cruise crew member, Allison, offered help and guidance. She gave me all the pros and cons of the life and hooked me up with the Canadian recruiter. With a good resumé and many years of experience working in arts administration, I scored an interview quickly. After a dozen questions, the recruiter told me I would be a good fit and she would be in touch.

After just a couple of weeks, she contacted me to say she

had secured a position in the arts and entertainment division as a cruise program administrator, or CPA, with Royal Caribbean Cruises. She assured me that the first two weeks were the worst but that it got better. She then reminded me to try to stay on board for at least six weeks before bailing so she would be paid for the recruitment.

I quit my beloved music-industry job, sold my car, and packed my bags. I purchased a plane ticket to Port Canaveral, Florida, to join my first ship, *Enchantment of the Seas,* for three- and four-day cruises of the Bahamas. (I would later learn this is not the ideal itinerary.)

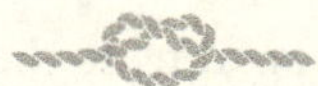

The cruise line put me up in a Best Western hotel in Orlando, letting me know that another crew member might arrive at any time and share the room with me. I knew I had to get used to this awkward possibility but slept anxiously that night, waking to every sound I heard. Luckily, I woke the next morning to an empty bed beside me so I could mentally prepare alone.

That morning, a shuttle bus picked me up at six o'clock to take me to the port.

Anticipating a hectic day with a lot of "hurry up and wait," I was excited and nervous but more than ready for the adventure when I hopped on the shuttle.

"New hire?" someone said while I found my seat.

"Yeah," I said, wondering how they knew that.

Like he could read my mind, he said, matter-of-factly, "You look like a new hire."

Whatever that meant. I quietly smiled and settled in for the drive to Port Canaveral. Maybe it was all the smiling. Or my style—or lack thereof. While the uniforms are hideous across the board, the crew have an excellent personal style when not on the clock. I felt somewhat out of place in my usual band T-shirts, flannel, and Birkenstocks, which I later learned were "crunchy white people" shoes. I didn't stop wearing them, mind you, but appreciated the heads-up on that.

When we finally arrived at the port, my heart skipped a beat when I laid eyes on the ship. I had never been on a cruise ship before, so standing next to her majestic size with my luggage, I felt like an insect. St. John's is a port city, so I've seen ships all my life. However, with its narrow opening to the harbour—coincidentally called "The Narrows"—rarely and only recently have huge ships arrived in port. While *Enchantment* is a much smaller ship than some of the newer vessels in the Royal Caribbean fleet, at 83,000 tons, she is still considerable. I was in awe of her.

On board a cruise ship like this, there is something for everyone! Dad gets to drink all day, Mom gets to watch Broadway shows, teenagers can go to a club, kids can play endlessly, and Grandma can enjoy the casino.

With all the new crew signing on, we had to file in long lines while our things were checked. We signed documents, got our photos taken for our IDs, and more. After hours on my feet, I was taken down the I-95, a long, hidden walkway that goes from one end of the ship to the other. Its secret passageways make it easier and quicker for crew to get around. We then went through a series of hallways to my cabin, my living space for the next seven months. I couldn't wait to get settled in.

"Drop off your things and meet me back at HR in ten minutes," said the hurried crew member, who quickly left me in the room.

I had no idea how to return to the I-95, let alone HR.

All the crew cabins are small, and unless you have "3+ stripes," you'll probably be sharing with a cabin mate. These rules applied when I was on board, from September 2015 to November 2016. The same-sex crew are always matched together, the nonbinary crew pick their preference, and any on-board couples must be registered couples to share a cabin. A couple must not only do a ton of paperwork on board; they must get married or share proof of address on land for an extended time. But ship relationships can be notoriously fickle, so it's not easy to get registered.

Each cabin typically has single-mattress bunk beds, a small TV, a minifridge, a closet, and a small bathroom. Most crew members get curtains for additional privacy in their bunk-bed quarters, which is a nice and appreciated touch. A cabin is typically 120 square feet. In comparison, the average hotel room is about 300 square feet. The bathroom only has space for a sink, toilet, and shower, and they're usually pretty cramped together, making the space feel very tight. The wet shower curtain clings to your butt, and the small space makes it almost impossible to shave your legs. It takes a while to figure out a method that works for you.

Although the room was small, it was a lot to take in. My roommate, whom I was told I would meet eventually, was from Peru and worked in Adventure Ocean, helping run the children's programming on board. Her bunk and half of the room were covered in stuffed Disney characters. Further, the room had multiple air fresheners, most on timers, that puffed out little smelly clouds of perfume. I wasn't sure if I was more worried about inhaling her perfume, which made me prone to headaches, or living with a Disney adult. Luckily, she was very sweet, and she and her air fresheners signed off shortly thereafter, easing my headaches.

This was my first Facebook post after settling in: *All is well! Everyone thinks I'm Irish.*

It seemed, particularly when I was on the back deck having some drinks, that people thought my Newfoundland accent was Irish.

"Are you Irish? What's that accent?" they'd say.

"I'm a Newfoundlander."

Some would give a blank stare. The eyes of others, mostly guests, would light up if they were in the know about our little island. "Ah, Newfoundlander! Newfie, right?! What ya at, right?"

The accent is tough to impersonate, particularly those charming and quick rural accents born of towns with a maximum of a thousand people living there.

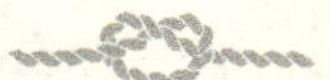

My job on board was an odd one. It was called cruise program administrator, but everyone called me CPA. It was, in a nutshell, administration for the arts and entertainment department on board. Every Royal Caribbean ship has one and only one CPA. I was "senior staff" in charge of all logistics for the entertainment division, including room assignments, scheduling, and the evil Kronos, which housed our time sheets.

In Deedee Presser's book *Shipwrecked*, she says, "You do not want to be on the CPA's bad side." Because I dealt with all the comings and goings of everyone from singers, dancers, and musicians to the youth staff, sports staff, and stage crew, it's true I may not have been the best person to cross. Otherwise, I had no authority and still had to share a cabin like everyone else. Luckily, since I assigned cabins, I got to hand-pick my cabin and my next roommate.

The CPA I was replacing was an Australian named Nicole, who sounded American. She told me she had lived away for so long that she'd lost her accent. She had joined ships as a dancer when she was just eighteen and had remained on ships well after she stopped dancing. She enjoyed the travelling lifestyle. It was clear to me from the jump that many people on board were intimidated by Nicole and maybe even slightly scared of her. It was crystal clear that she knew ship life inside and out and, without hesitation, was always quick to correct someone and provide the proper procedures. Even people who ranked well above her.

Nicole was a true professional and, looking back, the best teacher I could have had to prepare for crazy ship life. We bonded before she left the ship, and she was an incredible source of information for my job on board. (Thank you, Nicole!)

Between the job and rigorous safety training, I was inundated with so much new information that it was challenging to get everything straight. Nicole didn't have a lot of patience with me not catching onto things quickly and bawled me out a few times, something I wasn't used to, but I quickly learned that this military style was typical for ships. It was called getting a "banana," and you don't want that. I swear I still have nightmares of one director's incessant screaming.

On one of the last days of training, with a few people present in the office, Nicole started to give me a banana loudly. Embarrassed, I calmly reminded her that I was new and to try to have some patience with me. She continued for another few minutes and then introduced me to the ship's wig stylist, David. (Yes, cruise ships have people who come aboard simply to manage the entertainers' wigs). He was busily getting ready for drill.

"This one is good," Nicole told him with a slight grin. "She's actually gonna last." And then she bawled at him, "So you better take care of her, you hear me?"

"Of course," he said, cowering. He winked at me on the way out.

At that moment, I knew I had passed her test. I was going to be okay. I could do this. Likely noticing my out-of-place clothes, Nicole gave me a "perfect for our job" Calvin Klein dress because she "already had one in that colour" and signed off soon after. Wig stylist David did look out for me, and first up was my wardrobe. He took me out to buy five similar Calvin Klein dresses and two pairs of Comfort Plus heels.

By then, I'd overcome my anxiety about leaving the ship, or rather, about the process of getting off and on. Almost two weeks into being on board, I decided I had to get some items to nest, so a dreaded Walmart trip in Port Canaveral, Florida, was in order. I took a shuttle with some friends, and all was well until I got inside the building. I got land sick, which is the weirdest feeling ever. Being so accustomed to being on the ship and the slight constant rocking, I was walking around with my head swimming, even bumping into things from time to time, shaking my head to try to feel steady. My friend giggled at me, telling me it looked like I was day drunk in Walmart. Funny enough, I never once got seasick while on board. I like to think that's due to my islander blood.

I worked directly under the cruise director and the hotel director, doing whatever random task I was assigned by them. Different directors had different tasks and styles, so you just made whatever they wanted work. Apart from hours of administration per week, I would also emcee events, help or participate in shows, and assist guests with random requests.

While the first few weeks were, frankly, insane, it was soon apparent that I was made for ship life. I loved working and living on board and quickly found a close group of friends, who mostly consisted of the most beautiful Latino gay men you have ever seen. I started dating a Romanian casino dealer whose name I could never really pronounce.

Honestly, from the very beginning, I thought ship life would make the best reality TV series ever. There's a world of untold stories hiding below the waterline. Cruise ships are a floating gold mine of secret drama!

Because the space is tight and the pace hectic, the crew tend to forge quick bonds with friends and co-workers who become family in a short period of time. One of the defining aspects of cruise-ship life is the tight-knit community of crew members. With colleagues hailing from various corners of the globe, the ship becomes a microcosm of international collaboration.

Crew members will always identify each other by their position and nationality. You don't ask, "Hey, did you see Jane?" It'd be, "Hey, did you see Aussie Spa Jane?" From the engineers in the engine room to the performers on the stage, everyone plays a crucial role in the seamless operation of the ship. Being away from your home and culture can be hard, so you lean on the people around you because they are experiencing the same thing.

Even before I came on board, I understood that my funny-sounding mailing address might turn a few heads. Dildo, Newfoundland and Labrador, is somewhat famous for its silly name. It sits an hour's drive from the town of Come By Chance, which is just past Spread Eagle. The wooden oar pegs of boats were once called "dildos," and they say that Dildo was named after those. Now, of course, the word more commonly refers to something else entirely.

When I signed on, the HR crew and I immediately laughed about it; and like all things on ships, this funny hometown name of the new hire made its way around the ship in seconds. I was from St. John's, reared in the Goulds, but after trying to explain it was my parents' address a dozen times, I stopped. I took the opportunity to use the town's name as a way to connect with people, and it worked. In fact, it really worked. Crew members I hadn't met yet would stop and say, "Hey! You're Dildo, right? Nice to meet you, I'm . . ." It was great.

So great I started using it to connect with the guests: "Hello, ladies and gentlemen. Welcome to tonight's Honeymooners Celebration Event! My name is Jen, and I am from Dildo, Newfoundland, Canada! Yes, you heard that right, folks. Dildo."

Laughter and questions always ensued, and the guests loved it. Passengers would see me around the ship and scream out, "Hey, Dildo!" I would wave and smile while we laughed at the confused faces of the other guests.

During my first week on board, a colleague took me to a Caribbean party, and I was enthralled by the hot and sweaty crew members' dance-hall party. I had never seen anything like this in my life, and embarrassingly, was trying not to stare at the rhythmic bumping and grinding. I felt like Baby from *Dirty Dancing*. While the crew packed in tighter and tighter, as the "new hire" was onboarded, I started to get aggressively hit on by people. I had no idea how to handle my newfound "fame" and the culture shock. I wasn't used to being hit on a lot in general—men from Canada don't hit on women this way—so I would smile and try and be polite and not hurt feelings.

My Jamaican colleague reminded me this was not a time to be shy. "Speak up, Dildo! Tell them *no*, and don't apologize! Don't act coy. They will not leave you alone! You have to grow a backbone on board here, sweetie!"

My time on cruise ships helped me grow that backbone, which was very much needed. At the end of my first contract, I faced a huge fear and jumped out of an airplane. While skydiving ten thousand feet over Florida, an epically embarrassing photo of my face was taken as I exited the plane. This photo was so beloved by my colleagues that it resulted in T-shirts being made with the title "The Flying Dildonian." (Photos are available upon request.)

A few months into the job, I was thrilled to get a care package that my mom had sent to the ship. It contained lots of goodies from home. I had specifically requested Kraft Dinner and Lays ketchup chips, as I was missing those Canadian delicacies badly. (My love affair with Lays ketchup chips continues.) Mom had included a bunch of Dildo souvenirs, which I gifted to all my friends on board. They were a major hit. She also added a bottle of Screech, which I gifted to my new American roommate, Lacie.

Lacie roared at my sayings. With my accent laid on thick, she started to repeat them continually. "Whatta ya at b'ys! Giver!" Her name tag in our office said, "Honorary Newfoundlander," so it was only fitting that a mock screech-in ceremony would be performed.

A screech-in is a ridiculous traditional ceremony for non-Newfoundlanders. It involves a shot of Screech, a short recitation in our accent, and the kissing of a cod—on its disgusting mouth. Missing from the on-board ceremony, unfortunately, was the fresh cod to kiss along with Newfie steak, which is more commonly known as bologna.

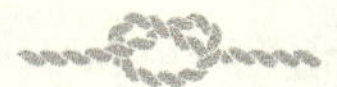

It has to be said that I was in a very privileged position on the ship. Like on land, the fact that I am a white, English-speaking woman from Canada makes me immediately privileged. The same goes for ships. That said, it didn't take long to discover that I was part of the minority on board the ship. Firstly, men outnumber women by about five to one. (Straight ladies, feeling bad about yourselves? Go work on cruise ships and reap the benefits of the limited pool.) Further, there were only three other Canadians on the entire crew, and very few crew members were from Western English-speaking countries. This was quite the culture shock for someone who'd grown up in a place with few to no people of colour.

Ship lifestyle combines adventure, hard work, and a sense of community. Working on a cruise ship is an education for those willing to embrace it. Crew members learn about different cultures, languages, and cuisines. They adapt to diverse working styles and develop resilience in constant change. The ship becomes a global classroom, offering lessons in both professional and personal growth.

Many of the jobs on cruise ships are filled with people from developing nations. One significant reason for this is that the cruise lines can pay them lower wages. When I was on board in 2015–16, the salary for most crew jobs was around US$500 per month. That included room and board. It's harder to convince people from the Western world to take a job for such a small base pay, but Filipino crew, particularly those living in rural provinces, told me that US$500 is the start to a comfortable life. In fact, Filipinos make up almost a third of all workers on cruises—and they work hard. Of course, officers, department heads, and those working on commission receive higher pay and can sometimes make upward of six figures. Traditionally, navigators and engineers are Italian, Greek, or Northern European, and many companies still have the usual places where they recruit. Captains are almost always white men, though Belinda Bennett made history when Windstar appointed her the first woman cruise captain in 2016.

Then there are the people who, like me, are privileged and chose a job on board not so much for the money but for the experience.

I also had a "side job" tacked on to my regular job. Luckily, it came with extra money, though not enough money for the job, I soon learned. I was the on-board wedding planner, which even included officiating for most of the weddings. When you oversee a family's special day, you need to be on your toes and ready to work. I wasn't prepared for how much work this would be. It was by far the most stressful aspect of my position.

The weddings alone were hard enough, in part because I badly wanted the families to have a perfect event. I had some great experiences doing weddings with some adorable families who were warm and friendly. I felt proud of those weddings and look back fondly on those special days. Of course, there were also couples and families who weren't as easy to get along with. Overly prepared brides with colour-coded binders outlining every detail they wanted were not the issue—I love a prepared bride! I'm talking about the bridezillas who were rude and entitled.

Cruise crew see the worst of the travelling public. I mean, just the worst people you have ever met.

One family got incredibly intoxicated the night before the wedding, and they all got into a fight with one another. Thanks to a zero-tolerance policy on physical violence, they were removed from the ship the next morning, before the wedding even started. Luckily, the bride was okay with moving forward with the wedding, because the groom, who hadn't physically assaulted anyone, remained on the ship even if most of his family and groomsmen did not.

I learned that one of my other couples had been married six times previously, to other people. That's right, they had both done it half a dozen times before. They were going in for number seven, and I was responsible for delivering their dream wedding. I hoped they would be an exciting, glamourous couple, but as soon as they arrived on board, the issues started. Both the bride and groom, who looked like they had stepped out of a *Trailer Park Boys* episode, started complaining about absolutely everything and demanding free upgrades and gifts. When I first met them, they were at the front desk complaining that their room didn't look like the picture online when they booked. Upon learning the ship was full and no upgrade was available, they grew irate. I tried to be over-the-top polite to the couple; however, it seemed nothing I did was good enough for these people. I just tried my best.

Their wedding was stressful, but I was relieved that it went perfectly fine. But then the couple started with their complaints, sending me a list of everything they thought could have been done better. Again I tried my best, addressing things on the list, starting with their first complaint that the photography wasn't good enough. I scheduled a meeting with the on-board photography manager and the couple. I knew how polite and likeable he was and thought it would be a great place to start. When the wife looked at the photo manager and told him, "I can't understand you with your fucking horrible accent. Speak English!" I knew there was no way to make these people happy. Let's just say the entire crew was happy to see those newlyweds walk off the ship.

As part of the job, I also had the pleasure of organizing any ceremonies or random events around the ship as requested by the guests. One of the most common was wedding proposals. I had some great proposals—lovely and moving—happen on the ship, and everyone enjoyed them. The entire ship would celebrate the couples, and they would cheer and talk about it for the rest of the cruise.

I also had proposals shut down. One man made arrangements to propose during the cruise's popular "Love and Marriage" game show, which celebrated married couples in the on-board theatre. When the man was given the stage for his big moment, the audience watched him grow uncomfortably numb, and the lady looked mortified. While the crowd waited silently, the cruise director joked to break the tension. But nobody laughed. I remember how loud her heels sounded in the theatre, clicking loudly in the silence while she ran off the stage. The man hung his head low and followed slowly behind. We didn't see much of that couple for the rest of that cruise.

Another gentleman on board had spent an obscene amount of money on the proposal he had planned for his beloved. I had to work with multiple departments around the ship to arrange the elaborate proposal, which took place in the theatre and needed extra lighting, a classical guitarist, fresh flowers, and so much more. When the day finally came, the department heads and I, who had planned the orchestrated event behind the curtains, were excited about seeing this woman enjoy her once-in-a-lifetime proposal. Instead, we all sat there, shocked, while the woman, instead of being excited, got very angry with the man proposing to her, speaking to him in Spanish. She screamed at him, slapped him square in the face, and stormed off the stage. The poor man, knowing how much time and attention the crew had put into the proposal, was so embarrassed by what had happened that he wouldn't stop apologizing—which was unnecessary, as we all felt for him. He even went to the on-board jewelry store and bought me a black cubic-zirconia tennis bracelet. The card said, "The gift of a bracelet the colour of my heart. Thanks anyway for all your help." At least he just had the staff watching and not all the passengers in the theatre.

Apart from the weddings, proposals, and my general administration of the arts and entertainment crew on board, I was also tasked with lots of random jobs. Twice a week, I was up on stage in the theatre, running the aforementioned "Love and Marriage" game show with the cruise director. I played a role somewhat like that of Vanna White on *Wheel of Fortune*, assisting the volunteer guest couples. We played the popular show in front of the rest of the guests, reciting the same jokes twice a week. (That funny answer you gave us about your wife? We've heard it a thousand times. It was said on the last cruise, and the one before that, and the one before that.)

Needless to say, altogether, it was exhausting. I hadn't napped since I was a kid, but now I was finding any spare time I could get to sleep. "Yes! Embrace the nap," my colleagues said. "You need napping to survive here!"

They were right. Passengers board with eager anticipation, and the ship transforms into a bustling city of diverse cultures and backgrounds. While those passengers enjoy their vacations, are the crew on the decks below enjoying their jobs? For the most part, yes! But that does depend on who you ask. It's no secret that crew work for seventy to one hundred hours per week, with no overtime pay, for approximately seven months straight without any days off. Vacations are unpaid. There is little to no work-life balance. You are pretty much on call all the time and live only a few minutes' walk from work.

When I started my second contract, I was informed by the CPA that I had a significant role in the on-board flag parade. The flag parade, which took place every cruise, was a favourite for the guests on board. This particular ship included a mind-blowing, face-painted Haka dance performance from my Fijian manager, Moe. It was magical. And no matter how many times I saw it—which was twice a week for six months—I felt it heavy in my throat, like I wanted to cry every single time.

Somehow, Moe learned that I wanted children but didn't think it was going to happen for me. He told me he could perform a quick Fijian fertility ceremony to help if I wanted. Just for fun, I said, "Sure!" For five or ten minutes, while I giggled, Moe hummed some words I didn't understand and did some hand movements in front of me, and that was that.

The outgoing CPA, representing Turkey, did belly dancing at every flag parade, and because the dance was allegedly one of the significant parts of the cherished flag parade, the position needed to be filled immediately. The flag parade represented the crew and all the countries we were from. Not every country was represented, only those for which the crew wanted to do a little performance. A Turkish restaurant manager performed in every flag parade and insisted on having a sidekick belly dancer. Since it was the outgoing's CPA's job, if I didn't do it, it was not going to happen. So I did it. Being a trooper, a Canadian trying to be a proud representative of Turkey, I strapped on a coin skirt and did what I believe to be the worst belly dance in flag-parade history, in front of hundreds of people. I think the crowd enjoyed my comedic performance, as they even threw some money my way!

Cracking up at my lack of shame, the cruise director told me, "The last CPA never got any money!"

It took me three weeks to find my belly-dancing replacement.

Speaking of shame and my lack thereof, as you can imagine, sickness—particularly gastrointestinal illness, or "GI," as everyone on board calls it—is taken very seriously aboard. All crew members are well versed in protocols, and GI happens a lot. I once got a very bad stomach flu and was confined to my cabin for almost three full days while I expelled the sickness from both ends. At first I was somewhat happy for the "break" from work, but I was feeling a little twitchy after two days, watching movies on my laptop and seeing no daylight. When I finally emerged, approved by the doctor on board—who some affectionately called "the Vet"—I quickly learned I had been awarded a new nickname. GI Jen. It was a glorious new nickname, and I accepted it proudly.

Always in my life, I have been connected to people in the LGBTQIA+ community, and my ship life was no different. I gravitated toward the queer folks on the ship like a magnet, and those fabulous men and women took me in happily. My posse consisted of some of the funniest, most gorgeous gay men on the planet—and strong, smart, powerful lesbian women. One queer friend, from Myanmar, will remain nameless. (I called him Smiley, due to his perfect smile and teeth.) There, queer rights still face significant challenges, and same-sex sexual activity is punishable by up to twenty years in prison. He struggled with hiding his true self from friends and family but was thrilled to join ships and finally live life as his true self—until he went home for vacation, that is. It was wonderful to watch him be happy, but so sad to see him post photos when he went back home, when his face was no longer so smiley.

It's not just the queer community letting their freak flag fly on board. Most of the crew are single, aside from the very rare married couple working on ships, and it's no secret that crew members hook up with each other all the time. There's a lot of sex going on within the crew—and I mean a lot. I saw several people come on board with a partner, and within a month, they were happily with someone from the ship. The tagline for ship life should be: *See the world, make friends, get laid!*

Consenting adults hooking up, being safe, and being themselves: fabulous! But of course, not all things are great about the ship sexcapade. I watched one too many wives get on the ship. We would all smile and greet them, knowing full well that their spouses had been sleeping with formerly virginal nineteen-year-old dancers for the past five months.

There was also zero tolerance for sexy times with the guests. Did it happen? Absolutely. We know all the nooks and crannies the cameras don't reach. The crew would also hook up in bars out in port, getting it on with guests who wanted to have a fling with an "exotic" crew member with a sexy accent—something to tell their friends about when they got home.

Hand in hand with the hooking-up culture is the drinking culture. If you're the sociable type, the crew bar is always busy. Drinks in the crew bar are only a couple of dollars, and people are there drinking seven nights a week, so you're never alone if you need to drink the day's stress away. I had been hoping to cut down on drinking, to make a change, when I joined the ship. But it was soon clear that I had gone from one boozy industry to another.

There is a policy that you can't have more than 0.05 per cent alcohol to drink, but if you're not sloppy or causing trouble, this is not strictly monitored. Crew members can't be intoxicated, but if you kept it cool and did your job, nobody cared. That said, if you made a fool of yourself or got into a fight one night while drunk, you would immediately be fired. During crew parties, everyone goes all out with the themes, costumes, food, drinking, and dancing.

Some of my most memorable times on board were those wild crew parties. You can be sure that guests would love to attend those crew parties. They ask the crew, "Where is that party sound and music coming from?" Under no circumstances were guests allowed in crew areas.

But for all the fun, there are also challenges. One of the biggest, when you're on a ship, is if you lose someone back home. In November 2015, I got an email—from the friend who'd gotten me on board—with the subject "Sad news from home for you."

She said, "You may have gotten another email in the last forty-eight hours, but I needed to send this. This is one of the hardest things about ships. You're so far away that there is nothing you can do with news like this. There isn't even really anyone to talk to about it. Your ship friends will care, but they have no connection to the story, so their empathy is limited. So, if you're ready, click on this link, and you will get the heartbreaking news. You will cry, so prepare yourself."

She copied the link to our friend Glen Power's obituary. He was a friend and drummer from my ex-husband's band who had lived just one street over from us, and we'd seen him a lot. He hadn't been sick but had unexpectedly and tragically passed, so it hit me like a ton of bricks. I immediately started crying and got up to go to my cabin, not looking anyone in the eye.

Later, when I emerged, I found a bag filled with chocolate hanging on my door handle, from a colleague. "I am assuming what is up, so chocolate for now and drinks later on the back deck if you are into it." I didn't even know she had seen me. Allison was right. My ship friends would care, and that was nice. That night, on the back deck, a large, diverse group of people took a moment to toast Glen Power.

While I did miss Christmas, birthdays, funerals, and weddings back home, there's one singular night that sticks out the most. I longed to be home for the final show of (arguably) Canada's greatest rock band, the Tragically Hip. I wanted so badly to watch with other Canadians on the ship, whom I assumed would be as devastated about singer Gord Downie's terminal illness as I was. But the handful of other Canadians on board were uninterested and busy running the ship, so I watched the beloved band play on my office desktop and FaceTimed friends back home instead.

After my seven-month stint on board, I went on a solo European backpacking trip, visiting Copenhagen, Amsterdam, London, Paris, and Dublin, and meeting friends I had met on ships in every city. I was nervous to do it alone but listened to Repartee's "Electric Everyday" for inspiration. I was hooked on the solo travel, and the trip was incredible. I couldn't wait to book the next one. When I started my next contract, my itinerary was to return to the Bahamas for a couple of months before heading off to Asia, then Australia, with plans to vacation in Newfoundland and then the Mediterranean.

Life was crazy and exciting, exactly what I was seeking.

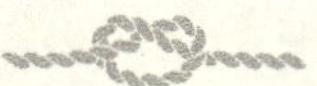

On my first day back on board from my European vacation, Canada Day 2016, I met Luiz. One of my aforementioned gay Latino friends—a Puerto Rican who was also Luis, but with an *s*—insisted on introducing him as "his new crush" right away.

"Jen, this is Luiz, Brazilian Bar new hire. Isn't he gorgeous?!"

Brazilian Luiz slightly blushed, said hello, and walked away while we all chuckled at Luis, who regularly enjoyed picking on his crushes. Brazilian Luiz was gorgeous. Even in his terrible uniform.

Upon having a drink with Luiz with a *z* later that night, I was the bearer of bad news: "Luis, I'm sorry to report, I really don't think this guy is gay."

"Sure, he is! He can't be that good-looking and straight. What a waste! Why do you think so?"

"Well, I'm pretty sure he was flirting with me. Maybe he's bi?"

"Game on, bitch," Luis said.

While I'm not known to be super competitive, two weeks later, I won the "challenge." On the back deck, Luiz and I stayed up into the late hours drinking, talking, and laughing. After a slow dance together, we kissed, and he started passionately moving his hands all over my body. I wasn't used to such a public display of affection but was very much enjoying myself, so I quickly agreed when he asked if I wanted to go to his cabin.

When we arrived on deck zero, the lowest deck on the ship, I stupidly blurted, "Oh wow, I didn't know there were even cabins down here." It was such an ignorant and advantaged statement that I was immediately embarrassed, but Luiz didn't seem to mind.

Later, after I had confirmed the rumours of Brazilians being amazing lovers, I asked, "So how old are you anyway?" I knew he was younger than me but assumed he was in his late twenties and told him so.

"Well, I'm actually 23," he said.

I turned red. He was twelve years younger. I was a cradle robber.

"I'm thirty-five," I said. "And apparently a cougar."

But honestly, I didn't care that much. He certainly didn't either. In my mind, it was just a one-night stand. Luiz was very handsome but appeared to be a little too cocky for my liking. (Luis, meanwhile, was not impressed, though he eventually got over it.)

Luiz and I continued to sleep together from time to time over the next few weeks. Although he was Brazilian and English was his second language, his English was incredibly good. He recognized and even used a lot of the same slang I used, and he seemed to like many of the same movies, TV shows, and music. One thing was for sure: we loved to talk and sometimes even debate with each other about politics or world issues. Oddly, we once got heated about whether Brazilians are Latinos or not. That one is still up for debate.

Weeks later, one hot and sticky day after working a long wedding on one of Royal Caribbean's private islands, CocoCay, I passed out after feeling dizzy getting out of the shower. When I woke minutes later, I collected myself and called the on-board doctor. My blood pressure was high, and I was a little dehydrated, so a nurse gave me an IV of fluids. Although I felt better, they asked me to return in a few days and check in.

In the days following, the dizziness kept happening. I was scared. I sat with a thousand-mile stare in my office, thinking about how my boobs weirdly hurt and felt heavy when I ran down the stairs to work that morning. I knew what that could mean.

In Nassau, Bahamas, the next day, I rushed off the ship—trying not to be seen by friends—raced to the closest store, and bought a pregnancy test. I then found the closest bathroom, which turned out to be a loud dive of a resto-bar, and headed into a stall. It took no time for those two blue lines to appear. And then I started to sob, overwhelmed by an odd sensation of excitement, amazement, and shock. I couldn't believe it. What I had fought so hard for and wanted so badly but believed I couldn't have was now happening. I found a quiet corner patio table and ordered a cheeseburger to get away from the partygoers.

Then I called my sister Lisa, who is twice over a mom. When I broke down into tears immediately, she listened and tried to calm me down.

"You don't know for sure what's happening until you get this confirmed by something other than a dollar-store test," she advised. "Try to stay calm. Get to a doctor right away to find out."

I returned to the ship and bee-lined to the on-board nurse. "I did a pregnancy test, and it was positive," I said.

"Well, that would explain your blood pressure." The nurse was looking at my reading. "You had past fertility concerns, correct?"

I shrugged. "Correct, but here we are."

She scheduled an appointment for me with a doctor in Nassau the following week, off the ship. I was shaking, sitting in the waiting room alone, surrounded by Bahamian women who kept giving me caring smiles, trying to make me feel better. With my face grey, nauseous, and scared, I likely stuck out like a sore thumb.

When I was in the room, the doctor didn't mess around. I wasn't his first crew member seeking confirmation of pregnancy. When he started the ultrasound, I stared at the screen, but it didn't look like anything.

He smiled. "You're about seven weeks along," he told me. "Do you want to hear the heartbeat?"

Shock. "Um . . . yes . . . I think?" I wasn't sure how to deal with receiving this news.

Then there it was, the faint but quick thump, thump, thump of my baby's heartbeat. And I burst into tears.

"Are those happy or sad tears?" the doctor asked.

"I don't know," I replied honestly. Never one to be lost for words, I could hardly speak.

The fact was, this was quite possibly the only opportunity I was ever going to have to be a mother. I was thirty-five and not getting any younger. I had actively tried to get pregnant for so long before with no success. Who knew if I could ever be so lucky again? I immediately understood that I was having this baby.

But I had no idea how I would tell Luiz.

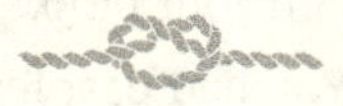

Later, I joined a Facebook group called "Royal Moms." The page was for women who had conceived while working for Royal Caribbean and wanted to connect with other moms from that cruise line. Each Royal Mom posted photos of their baby, listing what country they were from, what country their partner was from, what they had done on board, where in the world the baby was conceived, and on what ship. It felt great to scroll down the page and see all the ship moms like me share their stories. I wasn't alone. In fact, I was far, far from alone.

The stories of these mixed-nationality babies were sometimes beautiful and romantic, sometimes complicated and heart-wrenching—and sometimes both. Sweet families were struggling to be together despite cultural differences or financial struggles. Some women with children had never laid eyes on the father again. Inspiring moms displaying resilience and strength for their children against all odds. On and on they went. In fact, this Facebook group for just the Royal Caribbean crew had over fourteen hundred ship-mom members within the first year of launching.

My love of perusing the Royal Moms page got me thinking about all the remarkable stories that must be out there from female crew members from cruise lines all over the world. I soon became an administrator on the page. One day, it hit me while telling one of my besties, Allison—who was also responsible for me joining ships in the first place—about the Royal Moms. When the light bulb went on that these stranger-than-fiction stories would make a great collection, *Ship Moms* was born.

I assumed that someone had done this before. There are likely hundreds of books about ship life, right? Wrong. While there were tons of fictional cruise books, there were not a lot of non-fiction books from the crew.

I developed a plan and began scouring social media, and I put out a call for ship moms to share their stories. I posted on every crew page from every cruise line, contacted websites used by the crew, and emailed every crew member and recruiter I knew, asking them to share the information. Thankfully, the work paid off. In just two weeks from the project's launch, I had received fifty stories.

I set out to document the stories of these extraordinary women who, like me, had faced the challenges of a ship-life pregnancy. I interviewed the women in 2018 or 2019 and again in 2024. From the waters of the Caribbean to the bustling ports of Europe, the stories of ship moms from all walks of life criss-crossed the globe. What began as a simple desire to share experiences and find camaraderie transformed into a remarkable project that has changed my life and, I hope, has touched the lives of other women.

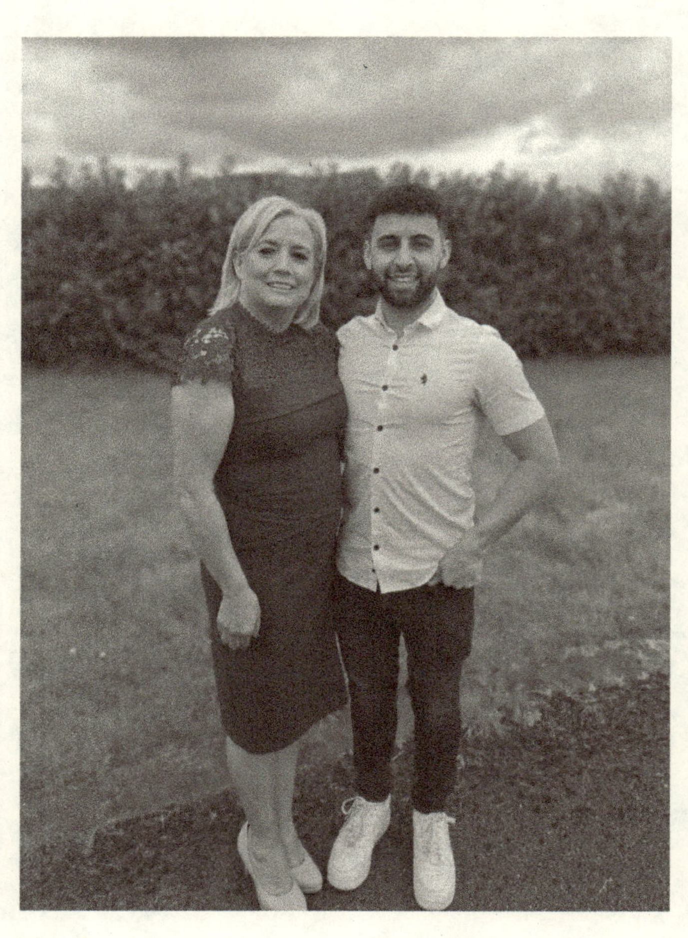

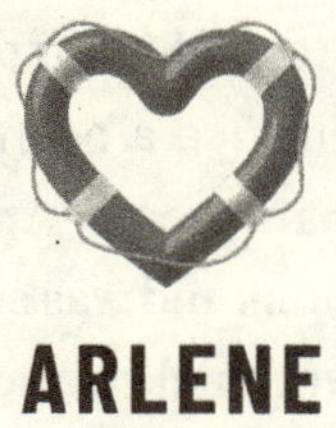

ARLENE

Arlene left her Northern Ireland community, population five hundred, very early to see the world. She started in her early twenties in Toronto, where she lived and worked, and in the following years, she made her way to London and Berlin. Back home in Northern Ireland, she was looking for a new adventure and saw an advertisement for Steiner, a renowned spa-services provider on cruise ships. It seemed like a glamorous life. With her passion for travel and a background in therapy, the opportunity was a perfect fit. Little did she know that this journey would not only take her to different corners of the world but also lead to life-altering experiences.

Like mine, Arlene's initial weeks on the ship were a roller-coaster, grappling with the challenges of adjusting to confined living spaces and navigating cultural differences in shared cabins. The job proved tough, and she thought of reconsidering her decision. However, the camaraderie with fellow Irish colleagues helped her find her footing, and she eventually started enjoying the experience and embracing ship life. She forged friendships and relished the unique experience.

Arlene enjoyed watching the on-board drama and intricate relationships. She tried to understand her extroverted roommate, who successfully juggled a boyfriend on the ship and a husband with children back home. Arlene acknowledged the prevalence of such situations and was astonished to learn about her roommate's unconventional relationships. She liked being involved in the party life but was more the type to watch from the outside looking in. The telenovela rumour mill on board spun all the stories of the crew during their maritime journeys, and she didn't want to be a part of that.

Eventually, Arlene met a handsome Trinidadian man on board, Sheldon, who worked in the casino. Like most, they met in the crew bar. He was friends with an Irishman on board, who had introduced them, and they got on like a house on fire. Again, like most crew, they got together quickly. They remained coupled up for the remainder of that contract, but because relationships on board are so intense, it seemed much longer. Arlene soon learned that he had a daughter back home, Lian, but that didn't bother her at all. Despite any initial challenges, they managed to establish a solid relationship. They discussed the possibility of a future together, but for now, they weren't taking things too seriously. When her contract was done and it came time for Arlene to sign off, they were so sad to part. They even rejoiced together when her replacement didn't show up and she had an extra week on board to spend with Sheldon.

Finally back home in Northern Ireland, Arlene was excited to tell her friends and family about her experience. They all knew about Sheldon, as she had shared stories of their time together, but not everyone got all the juicy details. Soon she would share it all with her sister, who was teaching in Spain. Arlene went to visit, and it was there that she started not feeling like herself. Missed periods were common for her, so Arlene was unsure if she had missed that month. Her sister joked that she needed a pregnancy test. She grudgingly did the test and was floored when it came back positive.

Arlene was shocked and scared. A million things started running through her mind. Geographically, she came from a tiny rural community of a few hundred Catholic people, and she was about to become the topic of the town: twenty-eight years old, single, and pregnant with a mixed-race baby.

Initially taken aback, she grappled with cultural and personal considerations. Despite reservations from her son's father, who cited career plans on ships, Arlene decided to keep her child even if that child was going to be raised in a community that had never had a person of colour before. She knew it might be challenging for them both but was ready to do whatever it took to make it work.

Arlene told her parents when they came to Spain to visit her sister. Her mother, always the detective, had felt that something was up and had asked her to tell them when she was ready. Arlene had always been a daddy's girl and loved her parents dearly. She had been scared of their reaction to her shocking news. To her surprise, they were happy and admitted that they'd thought something was really wrong, that she was sick or something. Her sister promised Arlene that she would be right by her side for any birthing classes or for the birth itself. It was joyous news, and with her family's support, Arlene knew she could take on the pregnancy and the world.

She told the soon-to-be father her intention to have the baby. Sheldon reacted much differently from her family. He thought first about his four-year-old daughter, whom he was supporting.

"Listen, I can't. I don't want to think of another child somewhere else in the world, where I can't be a father to them." He asked her not to go forward with the pregnancy.

Arlene was disappointed. She did consider his opinion, but the more she thought about it, the more she knew she wanted to keep her child. She had a good, supportive family and network, and if he didn't want to be in the child's life, he didn't have to be.

"You're going to be going it alone," he reminded her.

However, they kept in touch. Arlene remembers thinking how strange that was.

During the pregnancy, Arlene's phone rang one day, and a woman with an accent she recognized started in on her, demanding to know how she knew Sheldon. It was the mother of his daughter. She had seen Arlene's number on his phone and wanted to know who she was.

Arlene truly felt for the woman, who was obviously very upset, and tried to remain calm. "You're just gonna have to ask Sheldon," she told the woman. "It's not my position to tell you."

The day Arlene's sweet son, Anthony, was born, he came out with thick, jet-black hair and dark eyes. The nurses swooned over him, telling his mother, "Oh my God, he's far too beautiful to be a boy!"

Sheldon was back on board a ship but did check in with a phone call. He seemed happy to have a boy and called him "my son." He asked if Arlene would consider naming him Sheldon after his father. Arlene disagreed, but she did compromise and made it Anthony's second name. Still, a hormonal Arlene found his call confusing and upsetting, knowing there was no chance of a happily-ever-after. She had accepted her inevitable single motherhood, with or without the support from the father, yet Sheldon wanted the baby to have his name. He also wanted his son to have his last name. In Northern Ireland, anyone not physically present cannot be included on a child's birth certificate, so Arlene gave her son her own last name.

When Anthony was a year old, Sheldon's sister Georgette unexpectedly contacted Arlene and let her know she wanted to visit the tiny rural town and meet her nephew. Some of Arlene's family worried that it might not be for the best.

But Arlene, taken by surprise, wanted to be nice. More importantly, she wanted a relationship with her son's bloodline family. So Arlene was more than happy to have her come, thinking it would be lovely for Anthony to meet some of this family. Georgette stayed with Arlene in her home and even got to witness Anthony's first steps. Arlene's family remained cautious, finding it strange that his sister would come, but Sheldon wouldn't. Georgette stayed for a few weeks and often mentioned that she would welcome an introduction to any eligible Irish bachelors.

Sheldon occasionally kept in touch with Anthony with Facebook messages, first through Arlene. He eventually communicated directly with Anthony himself when the boy was old enough. Every so often, when Sheldon was close to that part of the world, he would mention he might visit, but would then give reasons why he couldn't come. "I can only stay for a week. It wouldn't be long enough. Let's try again soon." This went on for many years, and so, for many years, it was just mother and son.

Anthony's struggle with his identity as a mixed-race child in such a small white town was no secret to Arlene. They experienced double takes and whispers about them. In preschool, he was caught scrubbing his skin numerous times, trying to look like the other children. He was good-looking but visibly different from all his peers, so he initially faced challenges in school and the community for being different.

When Anthony was five years old, Arlene met John. She hadn't been actively looking for another partner but found herself filled with an overwhelming sense of joy around him. He was caring and protective, and they quickly fell deeply in love. She knew the meeting would be complex when she introduced him to her boy, but they moved forward.

Initially, Anthony found accepting the new family dynamics challenging, but he could see how happy his mother was. Soon enough, the couple was planning to get married. When John asked Anthony if he wanted to be adopted or to change his last name to John's, the boy said *no*. Arlene told her future husband she wanted to keep the same name as her son, to which John replied, "I don't care what your last name is. I just want you to be my wife." He was a keeper.

Not long after the couple got hitched, a new baby, sister Amy, was born. Soon there was another sibling, Lauren, a sweet girl with a rare chromosome disorder, and Mom had to be shared even more. Anthony loved his sisters immediately, and they were all very close, though Amy wondered why Anthony didn't call their daddy "Daddy."

John and Anthony never really had a warm and fuzzy father-son-type relationship. However, John worked very hard, six long days a week, to provide for his family and was an excellent father to all the children. He and Arlene worked hard to help see Anthony have the best college education he could have. Anthony could see that and was quiet and polite as far as John was concerned.

Anthony continued to keep in touch with his father, Sheldon, on Facebook, checking in from time to time. His grandmother, Monica, also phoned to keep in touch. Eventually, she reached out to Arlene and said, "I'm seventy-four years old, and I'd like to come and see my grandson before I die."

Arlene told her, "Of course!"

Since Anthony was in his teenage years, Arlene expected stereotypical teen behaviour, an "Aw, Mom, do I have to?!" response, but she was pleasantly surprised when he maturely said, "Oh, yes! I would love to see her! She can sleep in my bed. I'll have a blow-up bed beside her . . ." He excitedly started planning her visit.

Arlene wondered how Anthony would feel when his grandmother—a striking, dark-skinned black woman who wore a bright headdress—came to visit their little community. How would he feel about the turned heads or whispers? He made no mention of any concerns. He was so happy, and Arlene was thrilled because she wanted him to meet his grandmother—hopefully, on the road to embracing his father's side of his heritage. She wanted him to know his family and learn more about where they came from: their culture, and their traditions.

The following week, the grandmother called and let them know she was unwell but hoped to travel soon. However, she has never been able to.

When we first spoke in 2018, Anthony was my oldest ship kid, nineteen years old and passionate about music. He was hoping to pursue a career in music. He sometimes talked about going to Trinidad to see his Aunt Georgette again and to meet his grandmother and the rest of the family. He also mentioned going to Australia to meet his father, who lives on the Gold Coast with his new partner and works in bike racing. Financial constraints and the complexities of the dynamics, however, have hindered such plans.

Anyway, Anthony did not feel "abandoned" by his father. He has always been surrounded by people who loved and cared for him.

"The other day, after a few too many pints, Anthony spoke very highly of John and expressed a desire to repay him for all he has done," Arlene told me, grinning.

Checking back in with Arlene in 2024, Anthony, almost twenty-four, was still very much into music. He and his girlfriend were set to leave Northern Ireland in a few weeks to find work in Toronto, the first place Arlene travelled to when she first left home. While she will miss him terribly, she has always encouraged him to follow his dreams and pursue whatever makes him happy.

"Irish moms are renowned for being protective of their sons!" she told me. He will also be missed by his two sisters, seventeen-year-old Amy and thirteen-year-old Lauren, who Arlene says trust him absolutely. He is also very close to his Irish grandparents, aunts and uncles, friends, and music community. Simply put, Anthony is a special and very loved guy, and his big move away is a big deal for many.

Anthony hasn't yet made it to Trinidad to see his relatives but keeps in contact with Aunt Georgette and Grandmother Monica, who is now eighty years old. "Her greatest wish is to hold Anthony before she leaves this earth," Arlene told me. "I hope and pray this happens for both her and Anthony." A year ago, he received word that his sister Lian had a baby, so Anthony is now an uncle to a little Trinidadian girl.

Sheldon still lives in Australia with his partner. In 2019, Arlene messaged Sheldon to ask if Anthony could come to spend some time with him.

"Anthony was a little lost as to what direction his life was going," she said. "I felt if he met his father, it would help him."

Sheldon agreed, but then the pandemic hit, and the visit had to be cancelled. Last year, Arlene noticed on social media that when Lian had a baby, Sheldon and his partner had travelled from Australia to see his new granddaughter. During their travels, they stopped off en route in Amsterdam for a few days. Given that Amsterdam is only a few hours from Dublin, they could easily have invited Anthony to meet them. They didn't.

Sheldon and Anthony keep in touch, but they still have not met.

Arlene is now fifty-two years old and feels that as you age, you mellow. She admits that in the past, she had resentment and even anger at times, particularly in those special life-milestone moments. "The things in life that annoyed me once don't affect me the same way anymore," she told me. "I will be forever grateful to Sheldon for my beautiful Anthony. In fairness, he never made any false promises all those years ago. I got to enjoy so many precious experiences with my precious son in the last almost twenty-four years. It hasn't always been the easiest of journeys to navigate, and life always puts stumbling blocks in our paths. However, it's these experiences that help us grow the most. They make us more resilient and thankful for what we do have!"

Although I knew I was having my baby with or without the father's involvement, I thought about poor twenty-three-year-old Luiz. Rightfully, he had flat-out asked me one night if I was on the pill. I had briefed him on my marriage failure and how I'd never gotten pregnant before. Never had so much as a scare. I said I assumed it wasn't possible. Therefore, I was not on the pill. He said he was happy to hear that because the last thing he wanted was children. He told me his family had joked with him before leaving not to knock anyone up like his young cousin had just done. I kept thinking he would feel like I'd lied or tried to trap him. I didn't want this to mess up his life.

The next day, Luiz noticed I wasn't at one of the ship's crew parties, which was very abnormal for me, so he called my room.

"Why are you not here, woman? Come out!" he said, probably looking to set up his booty call for the night.

"I'm not feeling great," I said, not knowing how to respond.

"Oh? Maybe I'll come over? I know your roommate is gone."

I could practically hear his sly grin. I didn't know what to say but figured, what better time than now? My roommate was gone, so why not just take the opportunity and rip it off like a Band-Aid. While I knew he thought he was coming over for a good time, I was undoubtedly about to ruin his night.

When Luiz arrived, he knew something was up. I wasn't my usual silly self but rather solemnly sat on the bed, wrapped in a blanket.

"I need to tell you something," I said.

He sat down and looked at me, wide-eyed.

I didn't want to beat around the bush. "I'm pregnant."

Thankfully, Luiz didn't snap. He also didn't speak for a very long time. He just sat there looking bewildered. When he finally spoke, he asked to take a shower, which I thought was odd, but maybe he needed a few minutes to stand underwater and freak out without someone staring him down, looking for his reaction. When he came out of the bathroom, he looked a little more back to earth but still shocked. He then reminded me that he'd never planned on having children and this was not something he wanted. I thanked him for his honesty and for not getting angry.

Matter-of-factly, I let him know this was likely my only chance to be a mother, and didn't want or need anything from him. But I was going to have the baby. I told him I was signing off the ship soon, going back home to Newfoundland to be with my family, and he didn't have to worry or think any more about it. He didn't seem completely convinced, but he accepted my decision to move forward as a single mom.

My boss, the ship's cruise director, was very kind and understood my situation and my decision to leave as soon as possible.

However, I had to stay on board for a few weeks as the company made arrangements for my replacement. Luckily, the cruise director's partner was on board. Together, we conjured up the idea of her taking my job—perfect! I was happy that my leaving would make it possible for them to be together, and it did exactly that. They have since married and welcomed their first child. (Congratulations, Michele and Marli!) I packed my bags and handed over my job, anxious but determined to get home.

Nervous and stressed, my amazing ship friends helped me in every way they could during those last days, trying to cheer me up with silly songs, cards, and chocolate milk. My on-board bestie—a gorgeous gay Mexican man, Fernando—even offered to be the father of the baby one night.

"Tell your parents it was me! We had a little too much fun one night." He winked. "My family has money, and I would be proud to be your baby's father! I always wanted to be a dad!"

I thanked him profusely but told him he'd have to settle for "guncle," gay uncle, instead. Still, what an amazing offer from an incredible person.

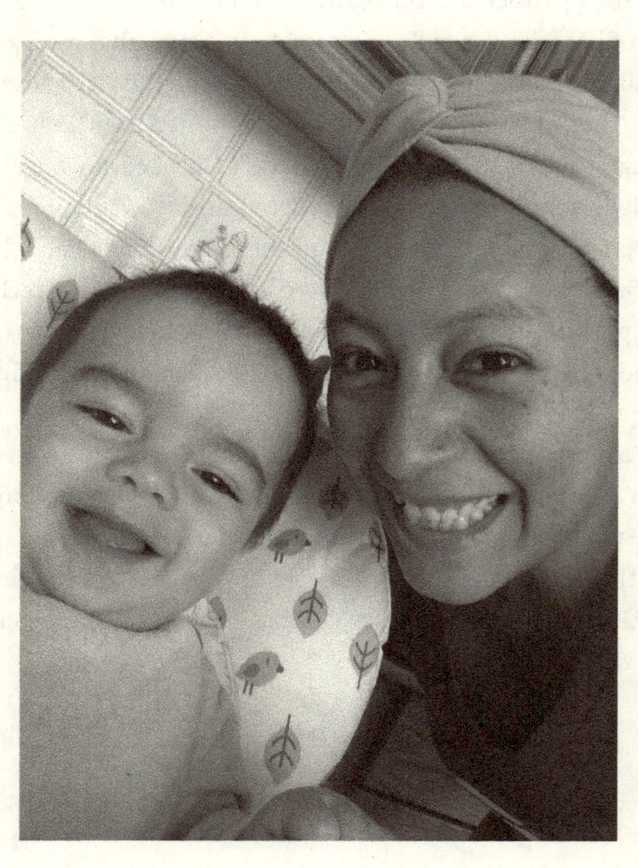

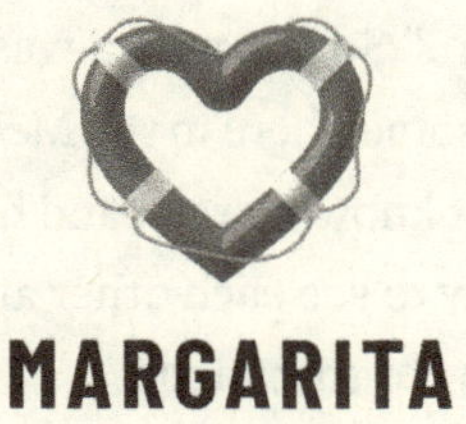

MARGARITA

A big fan of music and the band Queen, Margarita first noticed João when he was singing "Bohemian Rhapsody." His new four-piece band from Portugal had just come on board. It sounded so much like the recording and the singer so much like Freddie Mercury that she had to stop what she was doing and watch. The guests absolutely loved them and how they effortlessly shifted between genres and languages: English, Portuguese, and Spanish.

Later that night, Margarita was introduced to João at a cabin party with room-serviced wine and pizza. Musicians have it pretty good on board.

As a musician, João would do short contracts and would often move around, from ship to land. Margarita, who was from Peru, did six-month contracts, usually on one ship. As is typical when working on ships, they weaved in and out of each other's lives in different places in the world. They were acquaintances who eventually turned into friends. She loved his silly nature and crazy stories of times on the road. He was flamboyant and charming and born to be a performer. Her on-board boyfriend was immediately jealous of their closeness, and eventually let her know he had a girlfriend on another ship and that Margarita was the "other woman." So Margarita was single again.

On board the *Star*, somewhere in the Mediterranean, Margarita ran into João again, not knowing the band had just come on board. The friends were happy to see each other and planned to meet up for a drink in the crew bar that night.

"I love that red dress on you tonight," João said, winking at her.

She laughed at him, hit his arm, and rolled her eyes at the friendly compliment. Margarita had lots of gay friends on board who would say the same thing, maybe followed by a cheeky finger snap. But the way João said it was starting to feel different. Was he flirting with her? While they caught up, he told her how great she looked and kept handing her Smirnoff Ice, her favourite drink.

A few weeks later, they found themselves sharing drinks again. João brought a dozen or more Smirnoff bottles and put them on her table. Sitting down next to her, he said, "I bought everything they had. Did I tell you about my ex-girlfriend?"

Margarita was shocked to hear of an ex-girlfriend. João took out his phone and started showing her photos of the tall, thin woman.

"She cheated on me." João flipped through the photos, showing her every one of his ex-girlfriend that he could find. They both looked happy in the photos. Margarita found herself excited at learning that João was bisexual.

"She's beautiful," Margarita said, sounding defeated. The ex was Polish and looked like a model.

"She is beautiful, yes!" he replied. "So are you. She told me I was the best kisser. You should try my kisses."

She was surprised and was enjoying the attention, like anyone would. But ultimately, she thought he was silly and friendly and not at all romantic. He continued to flirt with her at every opportunity, and she was flattered by the compliments. He would constantly ask her to come to his cabin, and she would always say "maybe," with no intention of going. He enjoyed the chase and kept pursuing her.

While some women would be turned off by a bisexual man, Margarita was more open-minded and understanding, and she soon found herself starting to flirt back with João. She was going through a sad breakup with her latest love, an Eastern European man, and figured why not try something with João.

When she pointed out the ex who had broken her heart, João said: "Everyone makes mistakes."

She decided right then that if he asked her to go with him to his cabin that night, she would.

And so they ended up there, drinking and listening to music, learning that they had more in common than they had thought. Eventually, he kissed her, and in a blur of red wine, they slept together and passed out in a heap. The next morning, they woke up awkwardly naked. They giggled over how they'd just had sex.

"I don't know what you think, but I liked waking up next to you today," João said. "I think we should keep this up."

Margarita couldn't believe what was happening. She had never imagined being with João like this but figured there was no harm was in exploring it further. They started a relationship on board, to the surprise of all their friends. Margarita was enjoying dating a musician and the perks that came with it: going to dinners and shows and staying in passenger cabins. She soon forgot about her ex and her doubts about João's promiscuity and sexuality.

Her ex noticed that she was moving on, so he tried in vain to get her back. João had fun with the competition, and even after he signed off the ship about a month into their dating, he kept in steady contact with Margarita on Facebook and WhatsApp. He told her how he missed her in his bed, and they talked about how they could see each other again, how he could travel to Peru or her to Portugal.

She fantasized about them having an actual future and was surprised at the feelings she had developed. But João was a man on the move. He did keep in touch with her. However, when he noticed how strong her feelings had become, he let her know that he didn't want anything too serious.

"You're such a great girl," he told her. "But you know how crazy I am. You know that I can't promise you that I can be faithful on ships, right?"

Margarita was disappointed but didn't want to cut him out completely. She told him they could go with the flow and see how things shook out, secretly hoping they would end up together when they were ready to settle down. They continued to keep in touch, but as time passed, the romance started to fizzle.

Two months later, when she found herself getting ready to go out one night, her favourite outfit was fitting her very differently around the hips and belly. She went to the gym almost every day and was very fit, so she was confused as to why she had gained weight. She'd had a period last month, albeit very short, and hadn't had sex since João. So it couldn't be pregnancy, right?

Weeks later, she started feeling nauseous all the time and went to the ship's doctor. She told them everything, and they assumed she had a GI bug. When asked about her period, she wasn't sure but thought she might have missed her last period, so they did a pregnancy test. After a nurse administered the test, she leaned against the wall dramatically, looked at Margarita, and said, "Shoot me."

"What?" Margarita asked, unsure of what exactly the nurse had said.

"You're pregnant." the nurse replied.

On top of it all, Margarita also soon learned that her sickness was not just due to pregnancy. She had a uterine myoma, a benign tumour on the wall of the uterus, which brought the risk of losing her baby. Upon learning of this complication, the ship wanted to get her home, back to Peru, to safely have her baby. They signed her off and put her in a hotel room in Mexico for days while she waited for plane tickets. By this time, she was bleeding through her clothes and afraid she might lose her baby there, alone.

On top of that, knowing that telling her family and João would be hard, she put it off for a bit. Finally, she called her mom and told her. Margarita broke down crying when her mother told her it would all be okay and to come home.

Then one day, while sitting in that Mexican hotel room, she saw João sign on to Facebook, and her heart sank. She thought, *If I message him and he gets back to me, I'll take it as a sign and tell him. Alternatively, if I message him and he doesn't reply, I will also take that as a sign, to leave it be.* She messaged him: "Hola."

That was it. He replied automatically. "Hola amor!"

She thought, *Oh my God, now I have to tell him.* She told him to give her a call when he had a moment. Two minutes later, her phone rang.

"You seem so serious, Margarita. Is everything okay?"

She was so nervous. Normally a chatty person, she fell silent for a moment but then let the words erupt, telling him quickly she was pregnant, had a myoma, and it was a risky pregnancy. He quietly listened.

When she stopped talking, he said, "Okay. Well, I'm going to be with you. I'm going to support you."

He didn't bother to ask if the baby was his. He just knew and immediately let her know he had a home in Portugal and wanted her and the baby to move there. He promised to take care of them. This offer was lovely, and Margarita wished for a life that would see them all together as a family, but concerns played in the back of her mind. She was still going to get the flight to Peru, but they would keep in touch and decide.

Eventually, a few days later, she was given a flight by the cruise line. She made it home to Peru, and while it was a very tough pregnancy, her sweet baby boy, João Paulo, was born. Mama and baby were happy and healthy.

Margarita sent João photos, and he fell in love with that boy immediately. João constantly communicated and often sent complimentary messages to Margarita, like, "I'm so lucky to have you as the mother of my boy."

Four months later, Margarita and the baby packed up and moved to Portugal to live with João.

João lived up to all his promises, and life was going well. But things were not romantic. Although they were co-parenting, it was quickly becoming apparent to Margarita that they would not be together, which was tough. Margarita struggled with João's lifestyle and felt competition not only from every man she met through him but also every woman. The friendship they had built started to crumble, and they stopped having fun and chatting with each other. They slept in the same bedroom but weren't having any physical intimacy at all. She asked him to be honest and tell her if anything was wrong and if he wasn't interested in her. She begged him not to waste her time. He would shrug her off. She didn't know the status of their future, but she did know that he loved his son and that her taking the baby back to Peru was not an option.

The couple started to have arguments. One night, during the carnival celebration, João told her about his plans to stay out all night, and things got extra heated. Fueled by confidence from his mother, who had encouraged Margarita to speak up, she reminded him that he had responsibilities and a home that he needed to come back to.

He then told her, coldly, "I do not love you." He told her he had tried to make it work, but it would never work. Any dream of them being a nuclear family was gone.

The conflict took a toll on Margarita and on their relationship. They continued to argue incessantly. He started going out even more—drinking, partying, and hanging out with friends. Margarita grew more and more paranoid and suspicious of his relationships, which soon resulted in snooping on his Facebook account.

She got the feeling that his friends didn't like her. Some friends glared at her and oozed jealousy when around her. She couldn't help but read some of the messages and found some in which João had told his friends that he wished she would leave. She read examples of how his friends helped with lies and happily pretended he was with them when he was in other places.

Worse, she quickly learned that his friend group had given her a nickname. They called her Jane, as in Tarzan and Jane. Margarita, who comes from South America, was the brunt of a joke for them, a jungle inhabitant who can "swing between trees." The ignorant name stung but was nothing compared to knowing that even João himself used the name. The burn of him not even trying to protect the mother of his son was raw. She held the information inside for some time, broken-hearted, not letting him know she had read the messages.

Eventually, one night, he officially "broke up" with her over WhatsApp while sitting in the same house in another room, instead of telling her in person.

Having uprooted her life and moved to Portugal, she wished that he had spoken his truth earlier. Enough. She exploded and told him everything, what she knew—the lies, the nicknames, everything. That she was devastated and had wanted to be a family with him, but she knew that nothing she could do would make her dream a reality.

Then, overwhelmed and drained, she took João Paulo and moved in with his grandparents.

Margarita was in Portugal on a tourist visa. Although they weren't a couple, when the discussion of her leaving started, João begged her to start looking for work and stay in Portugal so he could be with his son. He even snatched and hid both of their passports. He informed her of this over WhatsApp, as he was still unable to have a face-to-face confrontation.

Later, in a letter, he let her know she should be grateful for everything he had done for her. Margarita was shocked he was so worried about her taking off with their son. She had no intention of leaving unannounced. She had too much love and respect for João Paulo's grandparents, who had taken her in and treated her with love, respect, and kindness. Yes, she was grateful for João's support, but she deserved a loving partner whom she could trust. João was clearly not that person.

When I talked to Margarita in 2019, she had decided to stay, for João Paulo's best interest. She had also decided to forgive João. Dwelling on his lack of romantic love for her was not helping anything. By forgiving him, she was slowly able to move on. In time, the friendship that had initially brought the couple together started to show signs of coming back. They would laugh together and started to enjoy each other's company again. Their boy now beamed at his parents, happy not to be feeling so much tension between them anymore. They decided it was best for Margarita to move out of her son's grandparents' home and back in with João. Their boy, now age five, was thrilled.

When I reconnected with Margarita in 2024, I learned she is still in Portugal with João Paulo and his father. During the pandemic lockdown, they were all quarantined together and helped each other through that challenging time. However, she did start to see a therapist to help her with their relationship. She had discovered, being around João so much again, that she wasn't over her feelings for him. He was very obviously over her. She had difficulty trusting him in general, so she told him she needed some help, and he supported it. She was diagnosed with depression and worked on herself. João even attended some sessions with her, to help her work through some issues.

Then João's sexuality came up in one session, and he didn't like it. Immediately, they stopped going to counselling. João feels that his sexuality is a non-topic and that nobody, including his son, needs to know about this part of his life. He says he will never be in a relationship with a man, so why talk about it?

Margarita had found work in a hotel spa and has started studying psychology in her free time. When we were chatting, she was enjoying some alone time—and the chance to sleep in—while João and their son visited his sister in Portugal.

Margarita and João continue to get along well, but there is still no romantic relationship. They have a good system where they can each have time for themselves while the other looks after their son. Margarita has started chatting on WhatsApp with a man she met in 2021, but neither she nor João has been in any relationship of note. She hasn't the desire to try to find a man and would prefer to spend her free time with her friends, going out for drinks and dancing.

Margarita and her son recently travelled to Peru to visit her family and had a fantastic time. Although João Paulo had only spent the first few months of his life in Peru, he has a solid connection to his family there. He loved seeing all his relatives and took full advantage of the warm weather. The family doted on the ten-year-old, taking him to shows, beaches, amusement parks, and more. He gets spoiled when he visits, and what kid wouldn't love that? He did mention he didn't like all the Peruvian traffic, which contrasts significantly with his quiet hometown.

Margarita sometimes worries that she isn't a good role model for her son, as their life is unconventional. "I hope I'm not giving the wrong impression to him," she said. "I want him to know what a 'normal' family is like."

That said, she acknowledges that while she and João aren't together as a couple, they show him how they communicate and get along well. "I want to show him a healthy relationship. Everything is about him and his happiness."

Margarita has started to investigate ways of moving out on her own. When she told João Paulo about it, he started to cry and didn't want to. João didn't seem too keen on the idea either, but she renewed her application to the government for housing support for migrant mothers again this year. If her number is picked, she will move out. She feels this might be hard initially, but eventually, it will be best for everyone. It's hard, she pointed out, to meet someone when you are living with your baby daddy, which is fair enough.

Although Margarita was once called "Jane" as a put-down, I wanted to remind her that Jane Porter was a charismatic ethnologist badass. Intelligent and capable, she was far more than Tarzan's love interest. She was a woman ahead of her time who demanded to be seen as an equal. Just like Margarita.

She sometimes wishes they could have been a nuclear family unit, but she's happy for what they have. As unconventional as it is, at the end of the day, they are still one family.

While I was wrapping up my last days on board, Luiz kept calling me, wanting to see me and, confusingly, acting like I hadn't just told him I was pregnant with his kid—a kid he didn't want. But the reality was, although we were just having a fling, we did enjoy each other's company, so we continued to hang out when we could.

Crew relationships typically fall into a few categories. First, we have the "hookup" relationship. This might start with a one-night stand and continue for a bit, but both participants know it's not a match. There may be attraction, but it stops there, and no one is reading too much into things. Secondly, we have the "contract couple." This relationship might involve some feelings, but both know its "until gangway do us part," and neither has any intention of continuing the relationship after they sign off. C'est la vie. You keep the memories and move on.

Then there's the "long distance" couple, those who have real feelings for each other, make plans to meet, and travel together on their vacations. This category goes one of two ways: slow fizzling out or turning into our next category.

Lastly, we have "the lifers," the couples who are so in love they'll do whatever it takes to be together. Normally, they're forced into huge life decisions to be together. They arrange their following contracts together or quit their jobs, move across the world, and get married—whatever is needed to make it work. I had no idea where Luiz and I fit in these categories.

We never really talked about the pregnancy, and it was hurtful knowing that he didn't want a future with me and the baby. But I pushed those feelings away, telling myself I wanted to get to know him more in my little time with him. I thought about years down the road, when my child was old enough, how I could tell them about their handsome Brazilian father and what he was like. I wanted to soak in as much of Luiz as I could.

Rumours started flooding the ship about me leaving, including a rumour that I had been fired. The truth is, people get fired all the time, so this is a typical assumption when people leave ships. By my estimate, about one person every couple of weeks was let go, and unfortunately, as an administrator, I was a part of this firing process. It was very awkward, sometimes heartbreaking, to monitor someone packing their stuff to leave the ship after getting fired. Some are quiet and calm, while I've seen others scream and cry and throw a fit. The worst were the ones who would repeat, "How am I going to feed my family now?"

I didn't care about the rumours or what people thought. I was too focused on getting off the ship and making a plan.

The on-board doctor reiterated that it was important for me to leave sooner rather than later. At the top of the list of concerns was a travel advisory issued for pregnant women not to travel to Miami, our home port, where Zika—a virus that can cause birth defects—was actively circulating. The warning came after fourteen people in Florida were found to have been infected.

Scared but confident in my decision, I called my parents to tell them the news. After I said the words, "I am pregnant," there was silence. I had expected them to be disappointed, but the silence scared me, so I timidly asked, "Are you still there?" Suddenly, they both started cheering loudly into the phone. They, too, had been utterly convinced their middle daughter would never give them a grandchild. They told me they would support me every step of the way, which they did. I immediately arranged to stay with them in Dildo to get settled.

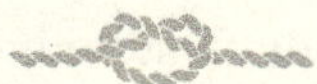

My last week on board was hectic, and I was thankful for my replacement, Marli. I had two weddings, which were challenging at the best of times, and found that my emotions were getting the best of me. Always the professional, I struggled through the weddings, overtired and choked up at times.

On the last cruise, a couple got on board and immediately asked to speak with me. I had nothing else on my schedule for events, so I assumed it might be someone looking to chat about a tour of the ship. The couple seemed nice and asked if I would talk to them in the centrum—the multi-storey atrium on the ship—so we slowly made our way one deck down to the comfy chairs, the man helping the woman down the large staircase.

The woman was clearly unwell, breathing heavily, so I waited while they got settled, assuring them I was in no rush, though I kinda was. The couple soon introduced themselves and let me know they were "from the south and not ones to lollygag." They explained that the woman was terminally ill. They wanted to do a wedding renewal and had heard I was the one who could make that happen. They hadn't gone through the traditional Royal Caribbean route to book their renewal, so I knew there were no booked resources on board available for me. But what could I say? I told them I would make it happen. We chose the last night of the cruise, during sunset, on the multi-deck walkway that runs along the ship's centre line, looking down at the pool deck on one side and the ocean on the other.

That night, dressed in my officiant best, I bumped into Luiz on my way out onto the deck, glad I was looking put together but annoyed that I was already flustered, getting ready to officiate this last-minute ceremony. I rushed past him, something I would never normally do.

When I reached the walkway, I was happy to see that the weather had co-operated perfectly. The sunset and evening wind were warm and magical. The woman now had a medical device delivering oxygen into her nose. The couple had recruited six spectators from on-board passengers who were funny and encouraging folks they'd just met and who made the moment even more special. The woman breathed heavily through her lines and joked with the new friends they had made, saying that they wanted her to hurry up so they could get back to the bar.

When I reached the end of the ceremony, my voice cracked when I said, "Please celebrate this renewal of vows with a kiss."

Everyone teared up when the very emotional couple started sobbing after their kiss. He quickly collected himself because it was making her start to wheeze. They were very thankful and took a lot of selfies with me, while the passengers hugged them and started on group photos. I said goodbye and wished them all well, giving the couple a basket of goodies with champagne and flowers I had saved. I will never forget this ceremony and how it felt watching these two people, so in love, preparing to say goodbye.

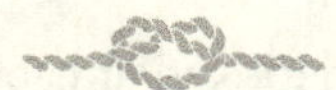

Days before leaving the ship, I got a call from Luiz.

"I've been doing some thinking and need to speak with you."

He sounded different. Confident but meek. He showed up at my room and confessed that one of our mutual friends on board had spoken with him, telling him to "shit or get off the pot." Thanks to my sweet South African sister Carmen, he had come to the realization that he couldn't have a child out there in the world who was his and not know them. He didn't know exactly what it could look like yet, but he wanted to be my child's father.

I was cautiously optimistic: happy but sure that when I was out of sight and out of mind, he would move on with his life, and I would move on with mine.

"Add me on Facebook," I said. "We can keep in touch there."

"Can it be WhatsApp?" he asked, a typical Brazilian.

Luiz came to my cabin, showed me how to get on WhatsApp, and helped me pack. That was nice because I had a large and hefty suitcase, a large backpack, and a guitar, which was the only thing I should have been lifting.

The day I signed off and had to say goodbye to ship life, my friends, and Luiz, I was emotional. But I was grateful that two Filipino friends who had also just signed off had agreed to help me with my stuff. Luiz seemed sad about me leaving, but I could never tell with him and his nonchalant ways. I was tearing up, hugging friends in the gangway and getting ready to leave, when I heard a crew member behind me huff and say under their breath, "It's just vacation."

Luiz and I hugged and looked at each other. I turned and left the ship, trying not to get upset and appear too dramatic. But I was dizzy with emotion. I honestly believed this would be the last time I would ever see my child's father.

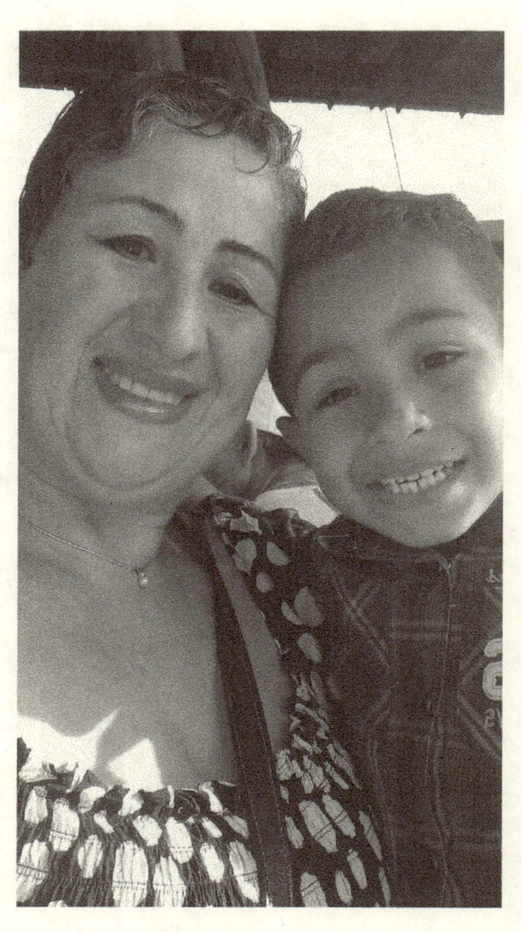

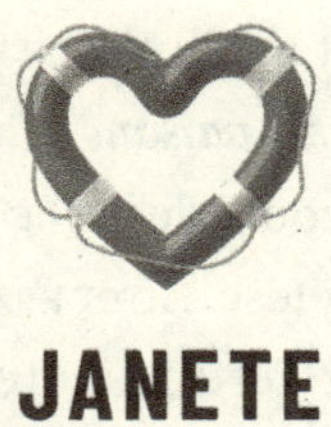

JANETE

Janete's departure from her ship was much more dramatic than mine had been. But like me, Janete believed she would never have a child. She'd been told "not all women are born to be mothers" by her doctor when she went looking for answers after two miscarriages. The sentence played on her. Obviously, she believed that she was one of those women. She would never have children. She would never be a mother.

Janete was Brazilian, a member of the housekeeping crew. In April 2019, she woke early to prepare for work, as usual. She showered, put on her uniform, and made her way to the office to get the master keys. Then she went up to the staterooms on the upper decks to begin cleaning. Suddenly, she started to feel sharp abdominal pains. Thinking it was likely just an upset stomach, she continued cleaning, but the pain was getting worse. Like all crew members, Janete knew the strict protocol: she had to go to the medical centre to ensure she didn't have a gastrointestinal illness that could spread throughout the ship. So she told her supervisor that she had to check in with the doctor. They both assumed that everything was fine and she would return to work again in no time.

When Janete arrived at medical, she was happy that the nurse on duty was her Brazilian *paisano*, Carolina. It made things easier knowing that she could describe her discomfort not only to a woman but in Portuguese. After assessing the situation and seeing that the pain was getting more intense, Carolina took Janete into one of the private rooms and gave her a sedative.

When the chief doctor was available, he quickly examined her and asked several questions. Then, the big question: "Is it possible you are pregnant?"

She told him about her past fertility issues and said it was not possible. He asked if she had been sexually active, and she said she had, but it had been too long ago for her to be pregnant.

"Maybe nine months ago?" he asked.

Janete went quiet while thinking back. During her vacation home to Brazil, at a restaurant in her hometown, she had met another crew member. Not a ship crew member but a handsome, foreign airline crew member. They slept together that night. Janete had thought that was that—just a bit of fun for a night, and she would never see the man again.

The chief doctor thought it was best to do an ultrasound. This was when Janete started to get nervous. She lifted her shirt so he could start doing the procedure. Looking down at her bloated belly, she thought about how much weight she'd gained since starting this contract. Maybe twenty pounds? Who knew? So, could it be possible? But she hadn't felt anything. Apart from feeling extra warm for the past few months, nothing seemed different. Her irregular periods had been completely non-existent for some time—which was completely normal for her—but for how long? It was hard to say. Ship life sometimes makes months feel like weeks, or in some cases, months feel like years, depending on your circumstances. She tried to remember the last time she'd had a period but could only be certain it was months ago.

The doctor put the cold goop on Janete's stomach and moved the wand across her lower abdomen. Immediately, there it was. Or rather, there he was. And he was not the little bean she expected. When she looked at the screen, she first saw a little face. Then a torso. Arms and legs. Fingers and toes. There was her son, who had reached nine months in utero and wanted out.

Shock is a dramatic understatement for how she felt in that moment. Not only was she unexpectedly pregnant, but she was in labour.

After the shock came fear.

At that moment, Janete didn't know if she should ask for help or just sit alone, worrying what was coming. All the things she hadn't done rushed through her mind. She hadn't taken prenatal vitamins. She hadn't watched what she was eating. She had no baby clothes or supplies. She was not prepared, emotionally or financially, for a baby.

She sat in stunned silence while the medical team huddled outside the door, whispering and using a tone that told her they were worried too.

They were worried for a very different reason. This was not a normal week on board the ship. They weren't doing the typical itinerary of a few ports of call close to shore and then back to the home port. Instead, the ship was changing home ports—from Salvador, Bahia, in Brazil to Tenerife, Canary Islands, in Spain. It was a transatlantic crossing that meant many days at sea. And when Janete went into labour, they were midway across the Atlantic. It would take at least two more days for them to arrive on land.

The medical staff knew that Janete and this baby did not have two days.

The chief doctor directed the nurse to call the captain and tell him he was needed in medical immediately.

Janete's English was not the greatest, but she knew enough to get by and have small conversations with the guests. She was picking up on the increasingly panicked conversation between the chief doctor and the medical staff. They spoke some medical jargon and exchanged concerned glances. Carolina rubbed her knees, held her hand, and gave her warm, reassuring smiles, but Janete could tell Carolina was scared as well.

Finally, the captain arrived at the medical centre. He took one look at Janete, and she could immediately see that he was worried too. He walked over to her, held her hand, and asked if she was ok. She smiled and lied and said she was. Even as she was awestruck by the captain's presence, she understood this must be a very serious situation.

The captain and the chief doctor started talking quietly between themselves, trying to find a solution. However, they were whispering loud enough for Janete to hear bits and pieces of the frantic conversation. The chief doctor didn't feel comfortable that the on-board medical equipment and team could safely deliver a baby if there were any complications. They decided it best to seek more help, so the captain asked that an announcement be made over the ship's main PA. They made a call to the guests on board for doctors, specifically obstetricians, pediatricians, and anesthesiologists.

After some time, around ten guests who fit those descriptions came down to the medical centre and gathered together as a team. The team examined Janete, then reported to the captain that they thought the baby was coming in about twelve to fifteen hours and that things seemed to be progressing normally. But there were some concerns, and without the proper equipment, there was no way to confirm that the delivery would be successful.

Soon enough, the medical crew were tasked with scouring the ship for diapers, clothes, and other baby supplies from any guests with small children on board. The guests were excited and happy to give whatever they could for the baby they thought was about to be born a few decks below.

The captain's wife had made her way to the medical centre to try and help. She came to comfort her stressed husband, who was scrambling to try and find a solution, but she ended up holding Janete's hand. The captain's wife sat with Janete for hours. She started massaging her back to ease tension, squeezed her hand extra hard when the pain came, gave her kind words of encouragement, and assured her that her husband was not going to let anything bad happen to her.

"We're going to take care of you. I will not leave you," the captain's wife said.

Janete felt relieved because she believed it.

The labour wasn't progressing as expected. It would seem to be moving along quickly and then slow down. Janete heard the team argue again about the concern of not having the proper equipment if a C-section was needed. She heard the captain repeatedly say he didn't care about costs or trouble. He just wanted his crew member and the baby to be safe. He immediately shot down any risky ideas, and Janete felt comfort knowing he was looking out for her.

After some time, he stood up and let out a long sigh. He shook his head, excused himself, and went to another room, taking the phone with him.

When the captain appeared in the room again, everyone was silent, waiting to hear what his next move was. The medical team started a huddle, expecting him to discuss the plan with them for approval. Instead, he walked past the team and went directly to Janete, lying on the bed, holding his wife's hand. He calmly sat on the opposite side of the bed, held Janete's other hand, and then took his wife's. Everyone in the room started moving closer to hear what was happening.

Peacefully and quietly, he looked at Janete and said, "I have requested that a helicopter come to rescue you off the ship. They're coming from Spain. It will take some time to get here—over twelve hours. They should arrive at around eleven tomorrow morning. The doctors feel your labour has slowed down enough that the baby won't come tonight. I believe this is our best option. Are you okay with this?"

Scared and confused, but wanting to trust the capable team assisting her, Janete looked to the captain's wife for approval. She nodded her head and gripped Janete's hand.

"Let's do it," Janete said. Hours passed. The captain, his wife, and the team took shifts, staying with Janete and talking to her, trying to distract themselves from the terrifying adventure about to happen.

When morning broke, everyone on board, including the guests, was aware that an emergency evacuation was about to happen. The crew was abuzz with concern for their crew mate, while the guests waited around the decks in anticipation of the rescue team's arrival.

Around eleven o'clock, two Spanish military helicopters appeared and hovered over the MSC ship. One had come to take Janete away, and the other was there to assist with the evacuation. When she heard they had arrived, Janete became terrified. She kept telling herself this was the best experience of her life, that she had always wanted to be a mother. And now it was finally happening. But of course it was happening in the most frightening way. She didn't know if her baby was okay. She didn't know if she was okay. She thought about the delivery and how much it was going to hurt. She thought about how her water hadn't broken yet and how that would feel. All the fears rushing through her overwhelmed her. She started to panic.

The team decided it was best to give her a sedative to calm her down, and she was appreciative.

The captain arrived to escort her outside. "Are you ready for this?"

"This is happening. I am ready," she said, convincing herself that she was perfectly fine with what was about to happen. But now she was feeling a little loopy.

Soon enough, Janete was moved onto a gurney and wheeled out of the room and through the I-95 crew hallway. The crew members and friends she passed in the hall reached out their hands to her in support. She felt better and normal for a moment, smiling at friends who reached out, telling her to stay strong.

But that confidence deserted her as soon as they got outside on the open deck.

The wind was whipping around, both from being out in the middle of the Atlantic and from the blades of the helicopters hovering above. One had ropes hanging from it, and members of the helicopter crew attached the ropes to a gurney, which had a basket-like contraption attached to the bottom. The team carefully strapped in Janete's legs and arms, making her feel both secure and claustrophobic. She was terrified, her eyes wide in panic. The only thing that kept her from passing out in fear was the pain in her abdomen, which had ramped up.

The captain yelled reassuring words to Janete, but she could only catch the gist of what he was saying over the wind.

The flight crew first tried to take her from the port side of the ship, but the winds were causing too much movement. Janete felt the strong gusts effortlessly tug and pull at the basket. Her heart leapt into her throat each time. The captain wasn't having it and demanded they move to starboard, so they did. The wind was still bad on starboard, but at least Janete wouldn't be in for as much of an amusement park ride.

The captain and his wife gave her a last-minute pep talk. "Remember to just keep breathing! Inhale. Exhale. In and out. In and out . . ."

Then they stood back and watched as Janete and the basket rose up off the ship and into the air. She kept her wide eyes locked on the captain for as long as she could.

Janete nestled into the gurney and tried to keep breathing as she had been instructed. Inhale, exhale . . . The pain was getting worse. More intense. She felt her whole self suspended in that basket in the air—swaying back and forth and turning around and around. Her heart was beating so fast she could feel it all over her body. The adrenaline was pumping, and she started to feel hot with sweat.

Then came a warm, wet rush between her legs. Her water had broken, and the warm fluid pooled up under her in the basket. She knew she just had to keep breathing. Closing her eyes tight, she pretended she was somewhere else.

Breathe in, breathe out.

To ensure the safety of all on board and to not distract the team from a safe evacuation, all the souls on board—every passenger and crew member—were mustered together on the decks like it was an emergency drill, which all crew members are rigorously trained in. Crew and passengers alike stood and watched in wonderment, taking videos and photos. Thousands of people oohed and aahed watching the helicopters and team evacuate the terrified crew member. When the basket was safely secured in the helicopter and the door closed, the entire ship roared with applause.

Inside the helicopter, Janete was scared silent. The kind and capable military medics talked with her calmly, letting her know that they had about four hours to reach the hospital. Janete had thought they were closer, but they were actually five hundred miles away. She could do nothing but lie there in the air and breathe through her contractions for a few hours—and hope that the baby wouldn't be born on the floor of a helicopter high above the ocean.

Luckily, they arrived in Las Palmas de Gran Canaria, the capital city of the island of Gran Canaria, in time. Two hours later, Janete gave birth to a beautiful, healthy boy. There were no complications. Without hesitation she called him Giuseppe, in honour of MSC *Seaview* Captain Giuseppe Galano, who had stood by her and stayed true to his promise to keep her and the baby safe.

The happy news was later shared via the PA to everyone on board the MSC *Seaview*, where the crew and the passengers celebrated the birth of the miracle boy named after their captain all night.

Janete was still uneasy and adjusting to the shock of what had happened, so she was very thankful to have been treated so well during her stay in Spain. A driver, Joaquin, a friendly man from the Spanish consulate, was assigned to her. He visited her every day to make sure she and Giuseppe were all right and had everything they needed.

Money had been a concern for Janete before—now she also had to take care of a child. Luckily, MSC paid for everything, including a first-class ticket for her and her son to travel home to Porto Alegre, Brazil. And the cruise line even let the airline know of the situation in advance and asked that she receive extra help. Janete was nervous travelling with the infant, and every time she had to present his documents, the response came with an eyebrow raised and a bunch of extra questions.

"So, you are Brazilian. The father is not here and does not know this baby exists. Your son was born in Spain. He's eleven days old, and now you are leaving the country with him."

"Yes, that's correct. He'll be naturalized as a Brazilian."

Odd looks, but she got the stamps and off they went.

Unlike his entrance into the world, her son was not at all dramatic travelling. Giuseppe was so calm and relaxed from Madrid to São Paulo that she spent most of the time just looking down at him in disbelief, smiling that she was holding a baby she hadn't known she was having. Nothing mattered then. He was healthy, and she was on the way home. Finally, the fear was lifting, and she felt incredibly lucky.

Meanwhile, Giuseppe's father was moving through life completely unaware that he had a son born in Spain after his mother, in hard labour, had been evacuated from a cruise ship. After Janete learned that he had more children with another woman, she was torn about how to approach the situation. About two months after she was home and settled in, he sent her a message on Facebook, saying that he had been looking around for her and was wondering how she was doing.

He must have seen her new profile photo with Giuseppe because the message ended with "And I see you have a baby now. That's nice."

She got back to him at four in the morning, when she woke up to breastfeed.

She said, "Hello, yes, and he's yours."

Of course the baby was his. Giuseppe looked just like him. He was surprised but had suspected it. The couple soon started a parenting arrangement. They don't have a romantic relationship, but the paternal family knows about Guiseppe and are always asking for photos of the boy who looks just like his dad.

When Janete first saw the videos of her evacuation, she broke down crying. She couldn't believe it was her hanging in that basket from that helicopter. Seeing it brought back the fear and the adrenaline of the moment when her water broke while all the crew and guests on board watched from below. For MSC, this was a first, and the captain told her that in thirty-nine years working on ships, he had never seen anything like it.

Janete is happy and healthy and lives to tell an amazing tale. She is so grateful to everyone who helped her during those few days but is unsure how to thank them. So many people were involved: not only the medical team and the captain and his wife but also the crew members and guests and all those in Spain who were so giving and kind.

When asked if Janete was in contact with any of the team members who helped her that fateful day, she excitedly told me that when Giuseppe was just a few months old, MSC *Seaview* was docking at a Brazilian port near her. Janete was invited on board so the medical team and the captain and crew could meet the baby.

"Our reunion was really cool, and we laughed at the whole event," she said of the get-together. She sent me numerous photos of herself and the crew members, wearing the biggest smiles and holding her baby son.

Catching up with Janete in 2024, I was happy to learn that she and Giuseppe, now five years old, are doing great and still living in Brazil. Janete is busy working and being a single mom. Giuseppe is thriving in school and loves going to the beach close to his home on sunny days.

She told me that his father had been somewhat present for the first few years of Giuseppe's life but hadn't been in contact for almost three years.

"It's all my responsibility now," Janete said, telling me that the relationship had turned sour during the pandemic. "We come from different cultures. We conflicted on education and religion, among other subjects. I tried to keep it friendly but could not."

Being a single mom, however, doesn't get her down. Guiseppe was introduced via video call to some of his paternal family, including his grandmother, which was very special. They hope to meet someday. Janete has also discovered that Giuseppe has not only one but seven half siblings from his jet-setting father—three sisters and four brothers, two of whom are also Brazilian. She hopes that they all get to meet someday too.

While Janete's pregnancy and delivery were not at all how she ever anticipated becoming a parent, she would not change a thing. She sometimes can't believe her luck and beams about how incredibly happy her little boy makes her.

She was born to be a mother.

To my surprise, Luiz started messaging me immediately after I left the ship. Always stoic and hard to read, he soon admitted to missing having me around, and my heart fluttered. I found myself staying up late at night, chatting and laughing with him, and I was constantly distracted by his messages. I quickly learned that, like me, he loved to talk. We'd chat and debate topics for hours, and I was turned on by his smarts. Eventually, we were in touch every day, all day.

I went to my doctor's appointments and watched husbands fussing over their pregnant wives. I felt sad but tried not to let it bother me. I went to prenatal yoga in sweats with a fellow pregnant friend while we made fun of all the Lululemon moms with their expensive matching outfits and perfect pregnant bodies. We would listen to the teacher tell everyone that our births would be as easy as "opening like a flower," which turned out to be a lie. We'd always leave yoga and get takeout, or what we called "second supper."

My sister attended prenatal classes with me, and my parents worked diligently to help prepare our soon-to-be home. Thanks to amazing friends and family, I knew I was not alone, but I was feeling down. I imagined having a baby with a partner in a loving relationship and not with my phone, which had now turned into a slight obsession. Like Pavlov's dog, every time the "ping" sound came from my phone, my heart raced. I craved the attention from Luiz badly. I wasn't sure if the constant communication was a good or bad thing.

We never talked about relationship status. It was beyond complicated. But we talked about everything else—and I mean everything else. We were getting to know each other well, and I was starting to really feel close to him. When he finally told his parents about the baby, it became even more real. I added his mother on Facebook and enjoyed looking at photos of a young Luiz, imagining what my son might look like.

I have an owl-themed kitchen—rug, salt and pepper shakers, sugar dish, trivet, and dish towels—and noted in the photos that his mom likes owls too. I recall Facebook banner photos of owls and a picture of her wearing an owl T-shirt.

Surprised but thankful, Luiz decided to extend his contract on the ship in order to travel to Newfoundland, to be there for the baby's birth. He was set to arrive three weeks before the due date. I was worried about playing house with Luiz and the feelings that would likely arise, but I still really wanted him there.

When I finally picked him up from the airport, I was anxious to see him, wondering what it was going to be like to be around him in the flesh and not on the phone. I was no longer the trim, vibrant party girl he'd met but rather a swollen and bloated version of her—full of baby and almost ready to pop. He was good company and wanted to help, although he admitted that he'd never held a baby in his life.

As the due date got closer, my blood pressure got higher. At this point, none of my shoes fit my ballooning feet, and I had officially hit the sixty-pounds-gained mark. I cringed at the thought of my swollen thirty-five-year-old body squeezing out a baby in front of the sexy twenty-three-year-old I was crushing on.

When the due date came and went, the doctors decided to induce labour, which went on for three days. I was anxious to get the baby out. On day four, I was admitted, and they said they were going to break my water for me. "A rupture of membranes will put you into labour," they promised. They were right. Contractions came hard and heavy, and I quickly asked for an epidural. Hours and hours passed, but still no baby.

After twelve hours or so, I was dilated to where I needed to be, and the pushing needed to start. Even with the epidural, the pain was overwhelming. I was lifting my body off the bed like a possessed demon, growling with the waves of pain shooting through my back. I kept pushing and pushing, but the baby simply would not come out. I was exhausted but not scared, assuming this was regular stuff. Until I noticed that my normally calm and collected mother, who had three kids of her own and had helped my sister through her two labours, had enormous, terrified eyes. At hour seventeen, my polite—sometimes to a fault—mother told the medical team they "needed to do something."

Finally, it was decided I had to have a C-section. Only Luiz was allowed with me in the room during the procedure. My body shivered uncontrollably with the drugs while they did the procedure on the covered bottom half of my body. When the baby was out, there was no expected cry of a baby, just a scurry of people behind the blue fabric wall.

I waited for the big moment when they'd lay my baby on my chest to have that first skin-to-skin contact.

Instead, the baby was whisked away.

Something was wrong.

I kept asking Luiz if everything was okay. While he didn't know himself, he kept reassuring me that everything was okay. But I could see the worry in his eyes while the medical team darted around the room trying to see what was happening. The fact was, our son hadn't started to breathe on his own. But thanks to the incredible team at the Janeway hospital in St. John's, he started breathing within a few minutes. Eventually, the team brought him out for us.

The feeling of relief was indescribable. Luiz cried when his son was presented to him. The tough delivery resulted in our sweet baby boy, Gabriel, having to stay in the neonatal intensive care unit for five days with an IV of antibiotics inserted on the top of his tiny head. To my surprise, Luiz was there the whole time and did remarkably well in that stressful situation.

Giving birth, I can assure you, is no fucking joke. I can admit now it was a traumatizing experience. Afterward, I said, "One and done." And I meant it.

But there was joy too. We were both immediately in love with our Newfoundland Brazilian boy, who we quickly nicknamed "the Newfzilian."

A few weeks later, on Mother's Day, Luiz left Newfoundland and returned to Miami to work on ships, which was like salt in a wound. I was mentally preparing myself to become the single mom I assumed I would eventually be. That said, we had just gone through a pretty dramatic thing together, and I felt bonded to him. We said we would see each other again when he was on vacation in seven months. In the meantime, I regularly listened to Yusuf Cat Stevens's "Father and Son" for a good cry.

Once back on board, Luiz stayed in touch almost every day, which I knew wasn't easy. By the way he spoke, I assumed that not many of his friends on the ship knew much about me and Gabriel but didn't push it. I noticed that Luiz never made any social-media posts about the birth of his son, so it hurt when he posted random selfies with friends. I started to wonder if we were a secret.

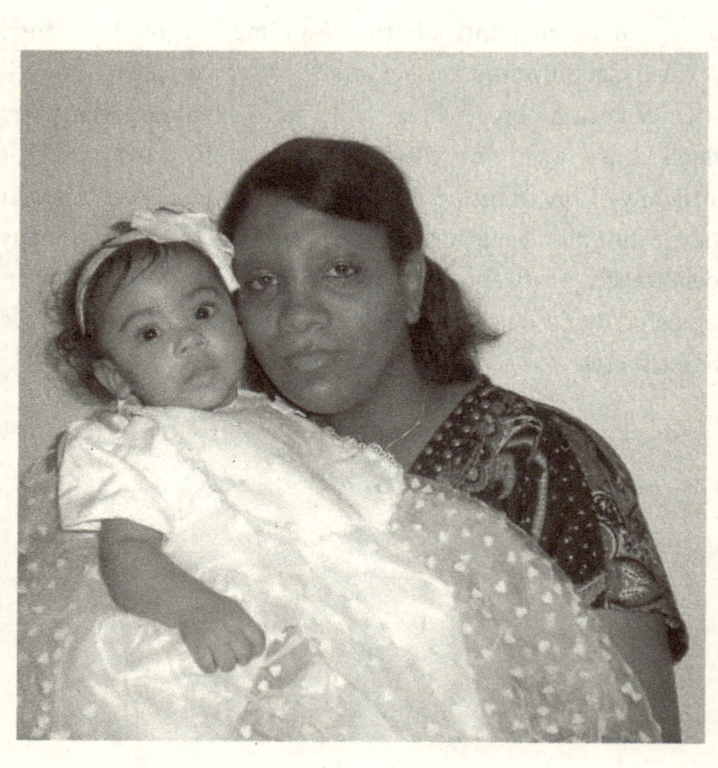

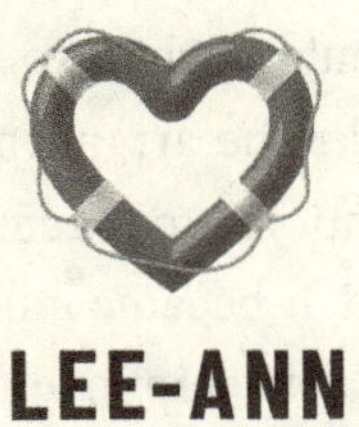

LEE-ANN

Lee-Ann was known to many on the ship as "the wise one," the one to talk to and get good advice from. She was the one who, when peer counselling a close friend on board, tragically witnessed the man die by suicide in front of her, jumping overboard just off the coast of Aruba. Lee-Ann and his on-board girlfriend had tried to talk him down, but he was distraught over the stress of juggling his two lives—his love on board and his wife and family back home. So Lee-Ann understood how much love and heartbreak can affect a person.

Lee-Ann and Nitesh met when she was dating one of his friends on board at the beginning of her first ship contract in 2005. They stayed friends but seemed to keep gravitating towards each other. She was an assistant server from South Africa, and he was one of many Indians working in the galley. There was something about him that Lee-Ann couldn't get enough of. At the end of her first contract, they started dating.

As with every new couple on board, Lee-Ann and Nitesh basked in the glow of their new "honeymoon" love. To make things even more official, they started sharing a cabin, which in ship life is the symbol of a serious relationship. In 2005 the process was straightforward. You would declare your relationship status to HR, and they would make the arrangements. But ship life can be complicated, and relationships seem to turn over like ports of call. So as time passed, it became much more complicated to share a cabin with your new ship love. In most cases now, you must be married or at least live together on land.

During this time, things were fun and light. Lee-Ann and Nitesh were in love and enjoying the time travelling and with friends. When they hit their third contract together, he started hinting at wanting a baby. As sweet as she thought this was, she was also focused on her future. She was working on her honour's degree in environmental geology online in her spare time on board. Her plan was to apply for an environmental officer position on board.

But Nitesh kept it up. He wanted a baby, and he wanted a baby right away. Lee-Ann was worried and thought there might be some agenda to this immediate need to have a child. She was focused and had ambitious plans, and nothing was going to sway her from those.

Nitesh eventually and somewhat abruptly stopped pressuring Lee-Ann to try to get pregnant. She didn't think much of this at first. She was too busy and focused on work and her future.

Then one day in 2008, Lee-Ann found photos of another woman in their room. She took one look at this mysterious Indian woman in the photos— which had obviously been hidden— and grew concerned that something wasn't right. Nitesh first said it was his cousin when confronted with "Who is this woman?" Lee-Ann knew he was lying. He then said the woman was his brother's girlfriend, since most of the photos were of Nitesh himself, his brother, and the woman. Obviously, something was off, but Lee-Ann didn't want to push it. She trusted him and loved their life together on board, and she'd never had any issues with him cheating in the past. So she moved on from the photos and didn't mention them again. They started talking about Lee-Ann travelling to India to meet his family.

Life on board was great, and they were happily in love—so much so that they soon got engaged. Lee-Ann had developed a relationship with Nitesh's grandmother during their time together. She was a hip and progressive granny by Indian standards and didn't want an arranged marriage for her grandson. She thought rather a lot of Lee-Ann and spoke with her frequently. His mother, on the other hand, didn't like Lee-Ann and told her in no uncertain terms that she was going to get rid of her.

Lee-Ann thought her relationship with Nitesh was wonderful, but slowly things started to feel different. The plan for Lee-Ann to travel to India was not talked about as much. She was busy studying and not taking her three-month vacations at home. Instead, during her vacation breaks, she was working on her thesis about volcanos and travelling to Alaska and Seattle to further her work and research. When she was studying, he was back home in India. During this time, she was focused on academics and not thinking about how her partner may or may not be spending his time. Their vacations didn't really match up, but since Lee-Ann was a manager on the ship and could make requests, she tried her best to make it work. That said, they always missed each other by a week or so.

Lee-Ann's focus on bettering herself and her education really worked out perfectly for Nitesh and his family's plan for him.

In 2010, Nitesh's hip Indian granny passed away. That was when trouble ramped up for the on-board couple and he did what can only be called a one-eighty-degree turn. He stopped communicating with Lee-Ann. Once, she'd known everything about him, and they had talked about their lives and the future. Now he didn't want to talk about those things—or really anything—anymore.

At the end of 2011, Lee-Ann and Nitesh were both a couple of months away from finishing their contracts. He had moved into a position in the bar department and was now working more nights. He had also started DJing the crew parties and had hopes of one day becoming the on-board DJ for the guests.

During one of these nights out, Lee-Ann was in the cabin on his laptop, which she'd helped him buy. He wasn't into technology and always said he really had no idea how to use the "bloody thing." She had taught him how to download music and use DJing software, as well as the ins and outs of using it properly. While poking around his computer, which was filled with music and all things for aspiring DJs, she came across more photos and videos. Again, that mystery woman. But in these photos and videos, it was very clear who this woman was.

She was his wife. The photos and videos were of his wedding. While Lee-Ann had been busy studying, his family had been busy arranging his marriage.

Not knowing exactly what to do, Lee-Ann decided to say nothing, to sit on it and give herself time to think. She wondered if he would ever really come clean and admit that he had gotten married during one of his vacations. She had known something was off, but had never imagined her fiancé had a wife in India.

Lee-Ann admits that, in the beginning, she was in a bit of denial. Her idea of what their relationship was had just flown out the window. Nitesh was already married and was living a lie. They had a mutual friend on board, Regan, who would occasionally tell Lee-Ann that he had to tell her something, but Lee-Ann hadn't thought much of it. She had been busy and working a lot in upper management.

Two weeks before they were about to sign off, Lee-Ann and Nitesh finally had a blow-up. She had been waiting for the right moment, but no moment ever seemed right to confront the man she loved, her fiancé, about his marriage. She started to talk to him about how they weren't as affectionate as they used to be. She asked him why he was avoiding her, going out all night and saying he was sleeping in one of his friend's cabins. There was something wrong, and she wanted him to tell her. She thought that he was cheating not only on her but on his wife, whom he never informed her about.

The fight got heated—very heated, to the point of almost physical fighting.

When Lee-Ann started to see red, she screamed at him. "Do you treat your wife in India the way you treat me?!"

He was shocked, silent. And then he cried. He wanted to know how she knew, where and how she had found out. He wanted to know if Regan had told her. Lee-Ann came clean and told him she had found the photos and video herself and that she had known for some time but had just sat on the information, letting it fester inside of her.

She brought herself back to when things started to change and how she had been so hard on herself, wondering what she had done wrong or how she could have thought things were so much different than they actually were. In some ways, finding this information was a relief. There was finally an answer to the questions that had been eating her day in and day out. This was also the final straw, an excuse to get out of this relationship and move on.

They only had a few weeks left on board together before they were about to sign off for vacation. They decided to stay in the cabin together as friends. With their history, it seemed like the best and most appropriate way to say goodbye and move on with their lives. She took the top bunk, and he took the bottom. They decided not to tell anybody about the breakdown of their relationship. They just wished for things to appear somewhat typical for the remainder of their time together.

For the most part, things were surprisingly okay. That was until a week or so later, when Lee-Ann found out that the wife back home had just had Nitesh's baby. While it hit her like a ton of bricks at first, she figured it wasn't her problem and started counting down the days until they would finally be apart and she could move on.

Lee-Ann kept her cool until one night just before signing off and leaving the ship, when she learned that her suspicion of him having yet another partner in the mix was true. Not only that, the woman—a security officer on board—was a hometown friend, engaged to a close friend of his. Nitesh had helped her get her job on ships to help pay for her wedding.

All those nights that he hadn't come back to their cabin, claiming he was DJing, he was in his lady friend's cabin. As it happened, this female Indian friend had started developing feelings for him, and it had become a problem. Hopeful that they could live their lives together, she was willing to call off her wedding so they could be together. The woman was all wrapped up in Nitesh and thought he shared the same feelings for her. But to him, it was just sex. He had involved another woman and was about to hurt her as well.

One day Lee-Ann accidently burst in on them in the middle of the act. Seeing that the woman was very embarrassed and ashamed, Lee-Ann didn't say anything. She could also see that real feelings were involved, and this is a major no-no in Indian culture. Lee-Ann knew the full extent of this complicated situation, not to mention that Nitesh and the woman were crew friends as well. Lee-Ann kept her calm until the woman had left, and then she laid into him.

"You are just finishing off with me! You have a wife at home! She just had your child! What are you doing!? Are you trying to ruin your marriage like you ruined our engagement?"

This would be the second time Lee-Ann watched him cry. He said that—ultimately—he had wanted to be with Lee-Ann but that it could never be, because his family had put him into this arranged marriage. He said he had an odd and standoffish relationship with his wife, but that it was also an unbreakable bond.

Lee-Ann assured him that she didn't have feelings for him anymore. Nitesh had hurt her too much, and she had moved on and was well on the way to getting over it. As soon as he'd started treating her differently, drifting away after the marriage, she had started to drift away too. She was done, but she told him she could be his friend. After Lee-Ann confronted him and talked some sense into him, he spoke with his lady friend and broke her heart. He admitted he was never going to leave his wife and told her to move on and be with her soon-to-be husband, his friend back home.

Finally, after all the drama with Nitesh, the time had come for Lee-Ann to sign off and go on vacation. She was excited about this one because it didn't involve studying and travelling but rather going back home to South Africa, where she could lick her wounds and vent to her family and friends. They hadn't been fans of her fiancé for some time, so this would be welcome news. Lee-Ann and Nitesh had travelled to South Africa only once in their relationship, which had spanned many years, so they all had a bad feeling about him. They were ready to celebrate his disappearance, and the vacation was wonderful.

When Lee-Ann arrived back on the ship, Nitesh was on board as well. However, they were no longer a registered couple. They got separate cabins and no longer hung out or even talked. They were living their separate lives.

In the crew mess one day, a fight broke out between two of Nitesh's friends. He tried to intervene and break them up. This backfired on him as he got hit in the head with a plate and ended up with a bunch of stitches in his head.

In a situation like this, all participants, no matter what, have to be reviewed in scary dismissal hearings. The two friends involved were fired immediately. As for Nitesh, the on-board management deciding his fate didn't know what to do with him, so they confined him to the cabin while they considered the outcome. Being upper management and well respected by the crew, Lee-Ann spoke on his behalf to the staff captain to help his case. Three days passed while they reviewed it.

With the uncertainty of his job hanging over his head, Nitesh was superstressed. The staff captain allowed Lee-Ann to talk with him in his cabin, to try and make him feel better. They had such a history, and he was going through a very hard time. While in the cabin, trying to comfort him, one thing led to another, and they slept together. She says a feeling overtook her, but it was just for the moment, and they said they were still friends. A day or two later, after a thorough review, the captain said that Nitesh could keep his job and stay on board.

He and Lee-Ann both went back to their happy and very separate lives, not thinking much about the intimate moment that had happened between them other than that they had both been caught up in it. This had been just a one-off moment.

Weeks passed. There was no talk of the slip-up in his cabin. But one day, the ship hit rough seas, and Lee-Ann felt sicker than normal from the rocking. She went to medical to ensure there was nothing wrong, particularly nothing contagious, and they started to do some tests.

Lee-Ann had gone off birth control after she and Nitesh had split months earlier, thinking there was no need because she wasn't going to be getting into another relationship anytime soon. When the doctor on board heard this, he told her they needed to do a pregnancy test. There it was. She was pregnant and not prepared, but she wasn't a teenager whose parents would disown her. She was a smart and strong thirty-one-year-old woman and knew right away that she was going to have this baby.

Lee-Ann struggled with having to tell Nitesh, thinking, *I'll tell him when I see him*. And then she didn't see him. And really, it was nerve-racking, so she didn't try that hard. Unfortunately, this led to her cousin's boyfriend, who was also on board, spilling the beans to Nitesh. He then waited until the end of her shift that night and confronted her. "I heard it through the grapevine that . . ."

"Yes. I am pregnant. And I'm not going to hide it."

Nitesh was upset, but Lee-Ann told him not to worry. She didn't want him to leave his wife. She didn't want anything from him. She just asked that, if she ever found herself really needing money, he help out if he could. She told him that if he wanted to be connected with the child, that was fine, and she would allow it. But she did assure him that she wasn't going to force him to do anything. He was angry and upset, but that was that.

Days later, she found out from a mutual friend that Nitesh was telling everyone on the ship he wasn't the father, that Lee-Ann must have been with someone else. He knew this wasn't true. She had been with no other partner at all, but for whatever reason, he didn't want their fellow crew members to know about the baby. She really didn't want much else to do with him at that point. He was agreeable to her face but then chose to deal with the situation in a much different way with his co-workers. After that, she pretty much avoided him, while he went on telling people that this was not his child.

It was hard. Stressed and exhausted, Lee-Ann started to experience high blood pressure. The medic on board suggested she leave early to take care of herself and her growing belly. She signed off and made her way back to South Africa.

When she arrived back home, she got a job at a call centre to make some extra money in preparation for her new life. About five months into the pregnancy, she started having complications. The doctor told Lee-Ann that her daughter was lying on her spinal cord, which led to sciatica. At times, she literally could not walk, which made her unable to work. The doctor explained how serious her condition could be for her long-term health and took her off work for the rest of her pregnancy.

Lee-Ann then knew she had no choice but to reach out and ask for a bit of help. During her pregnancy, Nitesh contacted her exactly three times and sent her money twice.

Sadly, she was in pain throughout her entire pregnancy. She developed depression and counted the days until the baby would come, in the hope that the constant pain would finally subside.

When labour began, she didn't know because she mistook the pain from her contractions for her regular, everyday back spasms. That night, when she got in the bath to try to soothe her aching back, she saw blood in the water. She immediately made her way to the hospital, knowing that her pregnancy was considered high risk.

When Lee-Ann arrived, the medical team rushed her to a delivery room. She couldn't give birth naturally due to the sciatica, so a C-section was planned. However, three other people were waiting for a C-section that night, so while Lee-Ann waited for hours and hours, she was given nitrous oxide—"laughing gas." Her back kept spasming, and the contractions kept coming. Finally, the doctor arrived and discovered that her water had broken some time before. She was fully dilated, and the baby was coming too fast to prep for the planned surgery.

Lee-Ann says she didn't know which were spasms and which were contractions, but she made it through, giving birth to her little girl while her cousin held her back up off the bed. When her beautiful daughter, Cheyenne, came out, it was like a switch had turned off. The pain was gone.

But there was another complication. The afterbirth had fused to Lee-Ann's uterus. After two hours of pushing, she had lost so much blood that her lips were blue. The doctor then went back to the regularly scheduled C-section to get the placenta out.

Lee-Ann loved her little girl, and they became an immediate duo—the two of them against the world. After Cheyenne was born, Lee-Ann didn't bother to contact Nitesh, and he didn't contact her. She posted some photos of her new daughter on Facebook, and they were friends, so she assumed Nitesh had seen them. If so, this would have been the first time he saw his daughter. She had the exact same birthmark on her right foot as he did.

It took about four months for Lee-Ann to fully recover from the birth and the sciatica. She had to go to therapy to learn how to properly walk again.

As well as healing from both the birth and the surgery she had undergone, she was struggling trying to find work. Getting back on ships would mean having to leave her daughter with her parents. South Africa has a very high unemployment rate, and because her scheduler had resigned, there was no longer a cruise-ship recruiter in South Africa. When Lee-Ann finally reached a new scheduler, she was told that her seniority had been reset and that her position on the ship had been cut. If she were going to go back to the ship, she would have to start from the beginning again, in the dining room.

With no other options, she ended up going back on ships. She was still having medical issues, though, and after another couple of contracts, she was signed off due to medical reasons. Cruise line companies cannot have crew with ongoing medical problems.

This led Lee-Ann to reach out and ask for help from Nitesh. She didn't want to ask but felt she didn't have much of a choice. And this was the first time she had asked.

He immediately got snappy with her. His response? "Don't make your problem my problem. You were the one who wanted to continue to be pregnant."

Nitesh told her that his wife had asked him to resign, that she didn't want him working on ships anymore. He was about to make his way back to India to settle down and be with his family there. He told Lee-Ann she was on her own.

She wasn't sure if Nitesh's wife, family, and friends knew that he had a daughter in South Africa. Frustrated, she decided to take matters into her own hands. She typed a long notice and posted it on his Facebook wall, along with a photo of the little baby girl who looked exactly like Nitesh's son. Lee-Ann also noticed that, because he was en route to Asia, internet service would be hard to come by, so the photo would be posted for some time without his knowledge. She doesn't know how long the post stayed on his page before he deleted it, but it was at least a few days. Long enough for people to notice.

The post covered all bases: how they had met on the ship years ago, when he had started wooing her, their engagement, and what kind of man he had ultimately turned out to be. She wrote in the post that she wanted to clear the air and let his family know about their sweet girl.

Lee-Ann was just content that the secret was out and his family knew. She received no feedback on the post from Nitesh or his friends or family, but a lot of people commented on it. Soon, all her Indian friends from ship life stopped responding to her messages.

Finally, she emailed Nitesh in the hope of getting some type of response. When he did respond, it was a written letter from him absolving him of any responsibility for his daughter. This letter was both a good and bad thing. It has been used ever since for any documents that Lee-Ann needs. Whenever she needs parental consent for something, the letter is an affidavit that proves she is the primary guardian with full and complete custody. There has been no communication with Nitesh since.

Cheyenne's paternal family members likely do know about her from the social-media post, but only Nitesh's brother became friends with Lee-Ann on Facebook. He must see the photos of his niece and realize how much she looks like his brother.

Lee-Ann gave the little girl photos of her father when she started asking questions like "Who is my daddy? Where is my daddy?" Cheyenne calls him "Pa" and says he's "over the ocean." That's simply why she doesn't see him. She knows that he and Mommy were together and that it didn't work out. But she has had some solid father figures in her life, like Lee-Ann's father.

Lee-Ann wishes she wasn't part of the majority of ship moms who never get together with their child's father again, yet she isn't surprised by it. She saw it a lot during her time on board.

When we chatted in 2017, Cheyenne—at six—could throw better insults back at her sixteen-year-old cousin than a teenager could. Lee-Ann's family always giggles over how the girl can be so different from the family at times. Lee-Ann laughs about how much of her father's personality Cheyenne has. She also looks a lot like him. The little girl inherited her father's way—stubborn with a quick wit—but she's also very intelligent and strong.

Lee-Ann told me that sometimes she feels sad for Cheyenne—though not sad for herself. She knows that, as things are, Nitesh doesn't want to meet his daughter, and that's what makes her sad. If he changes his mind one day, she will entertain that, but until then, she'll let sleeping dogs lie.

When I reconnected with Lee-Ann in 2024, I got to see Cheyenne on Zoom. At eleven years old—but "going on thirty," according to her mom—she seems all grown up but still very quick-witted and silly. As Lee-Ann says, her daughter is still a firecracker. She does well in school, gets good grades, and has many friends. She's artistic and driven and wants to sing or study special effects when she grows up. She's a very active participant in the School of Rock music school, singing in a band an hour's drive from their home.

Lee-Ann continues to live in South Africa, working hard in a law firm to support her family. She told me that she had just completed the business registration to start their own School of Rock franchise in their city. They plan to open the doors for students in 2026. It's not cheap; she has a lot of work ahead with the franchise finance and leasing fees and the plan to own the building and not rent. Lee-Ann said that this school will be a non-profit School of Rock branch, offering free music classes for local underprivileged youth. But she has also considered moving to Canada later on so that Cheyenne can access a better education.

They still have no contact with Nitesh; he has never met his daughter. He hasn't helped out financially or otherwise. Nor do they have contact with his family. Lee-Ann isn't sure if Cheyenne has any more siblings. Nitesh started following her on Instagram, but she rarely uses that platform. He did not send a message.

Using pictures of her father, Cheyenne has created an art project on a bristol board, written all in Hindi. She also shares her Indian side every heritage day. I wonder what her father and their family would think if they knew that this sweet girl he helped make celebrates his heritage and culture in South Africa.

Lee-Ann says she will be supportive of her daughter if she wants to meet her father and her Indian family when she's old enough to do so.

Although Lee-Ann doesn't follow Nitesh, she sometimes sees him on Facebook because they have mutual friends on social media. These days, she has no interest in reaching out to him or his family.

I understand Lee-Ann's difficulty letting go of her baby daddy—and how easy social media makes it to hang on. At home with my baby, feeling dispirited and needy, I started creeping Luiz and everyone he added on his social media while on board—particularly the young girls with gorgeous, perfect young faces and bodies. This was, of course, incredibly unhealthy, but I couldn't help myself. I tortured myself, assuming that Luiz was getting his rocks off with everyone he added to his social media. Every time he liked someone's photo or posted about his day, I grew more suspicious about what was happening on board.

Mother flamingos, due to stress and the demands of motherhood, temporarily lose their vibrant pink colour while raising their young. I felt like a flamingo losing my brightness. I wanted to get my pink back.

Apart from my social media creeping, I was content playing the single-mom role but was anxious to be around adults again.

Continuing to work in the arts, I started getting motivated and inspired by the artists, writers, and colleagues around me. I started actively immersing myself in new experiences and reading ferociously, which helped me reflect on my own life and emotional state. As the weeks passed, I started to feel more like myself again as my body and hormones adjusted to the new normal. Slowly, I began not needing Luiz and his attention as much, and he could tell. I was getting some of my confidence back again but still had a major soft spot for Gabriel's father.

At this point, I made our relationship status a topic of conversation. I knew what ship life was like and assumed Luiz was sleeping with women on the ship. My loud intuition bells frustrated me, but every time I hinted at it, he would tell me I was paranoid.

One day I finally told him that I was interested in discussing an open relationship because I was craving some companionship.

He wasn't interested. "I have you, and you have me," he said.

Thinking it would be good for us both, I planned a trip for Gabriel and I to take a cruise on Luiz's ship, to visit him. But before I was set to leave, I got a message from him: "I'm quitting ship life and coming to Canada to be with you guys."

Cautiously optimistic, I cancelled the cruise and prepped for his arrival. Looking back, I'm thankful he saved me from the embarrassment of going on board and meeting crew members who knew about things about Luiz that I was yet to learn.

When I picked him up at the airport this time, things felt a little different. I was no longer anxious but rather hopeful. I felt better about myself and more self-assured. By quitting his job and moving to Canada to be with us, he was making some massive sacrifices, and I acknowledged that.

Luiz quickly fit into my life like a glove, and we got along like a house on fire. Not to mention, the help with the baby was so lovely. It took no time before we felt like a real family, and I was beaming. Everything seemed perfect, but something was bubbling under the surface.

Weeks after he arrived, while we were sitting in a McDonald's drive-thru, I made a joke about other women on the cruise ship. When I looked over at him, the look on his face told me I was about to get hit with something. It was then that he confessed to being with another woman. While this obviously stung, the information wasn't a huge shock to me. I had assumed this but could tell there was something else. He wasn't giving me the full story. Over the following days, I drilled him for information—as people oddly tend to do when learning such news.

Who? What? When? Where? Why?

Soon he admitted to being with another woman. And then another. And another . . . .

I was unsure what to do with the information because, deep down, I already knew it. He had only confirmed it. I started to learn that what I had conjured up in my head—a worst-case scenario—had turned out to be true. I don't know how many women there were. I labelled the women he was with to dehumanize them, referring to them as "the guest," "the photographer," "the Ukrainian," and whatnot. None hurt more than when I learned that he had been in an ongoing sexual relationship with a Brazilian *paisano* of his, who—interestingly enough—was also in her midthirties. He started seeing her after our son was born and had even sent me selfies of himself and his "good friend." The Brazilian woman knew about me and the baby, but thought we weren't together.

When Luiz arrived in Canada, he gave Gabriel gifts that this woman had kindly bought for him. Not knowing the truth, I had thought it was such a nice gesture and asked Luiz to thank her. On board, the woman had also developed feelings for him. She even forgave him after she watched him make out with a dancer on board one night. She continued to send him messages after he was in Canada with me.

The moment I learned of this particular woman and the extent of the relationship, I saw red and went into a rage. I threw his phone into the sink, breaking some dishes inside. And when I saw the look on his face—his concern that his precious phone might be broken—I scooped it out of the sink, marched into my backyard, to the small river behind my house, and tossed his phone in the water. He watched it float downstream.

I felt silly and regretted it immediately, but in the moment, it was satisfying.

Then I sent the woman a nasty message on Facebook telling her she had ruined our family, which I thoroughly regret. She didn't know about the situation and was likely dealing with her own heartbreak.

I spent months trying to decide what to do while Luiz was making it very clear he wanted to be a family and was standing by. He remained with us but stayed in the spare bedroom. Part of me wanted to forgive him and move on, but I was still hung up on the betrayal. I childishly went all-out drinking a few nights out of spite. Unwavering, Luiz stayed helpful, patient, thoughtful, and kind, and soon, my coldness started to warm up. After all, Luiz was a young, single, attractive man who had sowed his wild oats on board. But he had also made major sacrifices to be with us.

Thanks to Luiz's tenacity—pushing me to constantly try communicating my feelings to him—I slowly but surely started talking to him again. Soon we were even laughing again.

This certainly didn't happen overnight. It took time, patience, and grace to move forward. He later confessed that I wasn't only the first person he'd had sex with on ships but also just the second person he'd ever had sex with ever. Growing up, he had been very thin and hadn't gotten a ton of attention from women, like he was now accustomed to.

It was clear that many stars had had to align when we got together and Gabriel was conceived. Even if we weren't going to be a nuclear family, our sweet boy was simply meant to be.

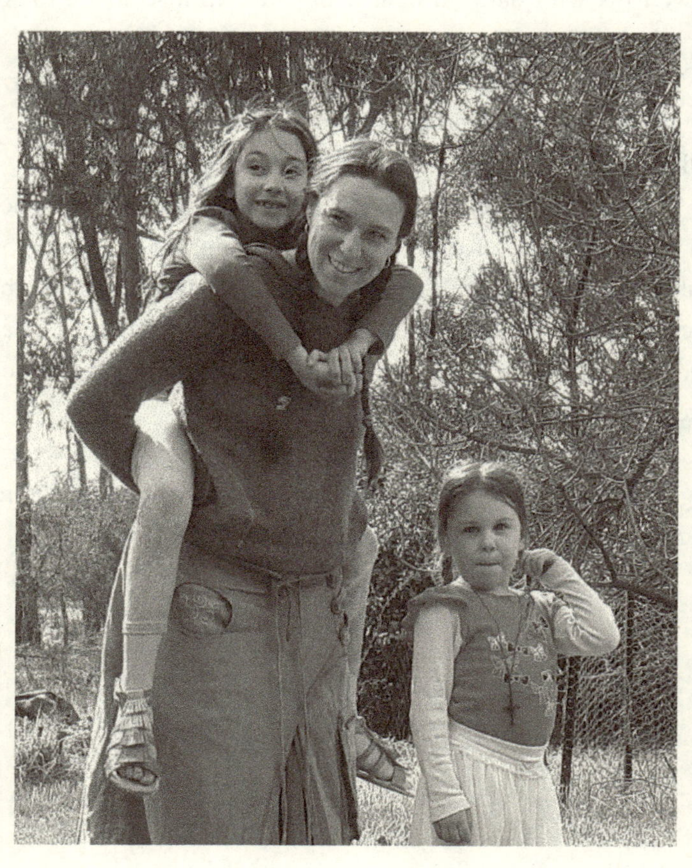

TANYA

While visiting her parents in New York, Australian photographer Tanya took a chance and travelled upstate to a head office for recruiters. When she asked for a job on board cruise ships, it must have been the right place and time. They hired her. This new job would start a significant new chapter and lead to a profound love that would change the rest of her life.

An extroverted type of person who loved to have a drink, Tanya was told by the recruiter that ship life would suit her. After getting settled, she found that it certainly did.

Boarding her ship in New Orleans, Tanya first met Rishi, a security officer from Nepal. Like most, as usual, they met formally at the crew bar and hit it off. Friendship blossomed, but they both knew from the start there was more, a camaraderie marked by an unspoken acknowledgment of the feelings that lay beneath the surface.

Rishi was honest with her: he had a wife and family at home in Nepal. Eventually, he also let Tanya know he was falling for her. She couldn't help but admit she was falling for him too. She was reluctant to be close and intimate, but these type of relationships are very common on ships, so she eventually gave in to temptation. Their undeniable connection grew into a profound love affair. In their moments of shared intimacy, Rishi and Tanya dubbed themselves a "couple made in the stars," envisioning a future illuminated by the brightness of their shared dreams.

The journey took an unexpected turn as reality had a different script in store for them. After her ship arrived in Malta one day, Tanya was hit with the realization that she might be a couple of days late with her period. A pregnancy test confirmed her suspicions, and the weight of the situation hit her so hard that she had to sit down to avoid falling over. The feeling of having made a colossal mistake overwhelmed her as she grappled with the implications of impending motherhood.

Amidst the emotions, there was a glimmer of hope. She believed in the possibility of a fairy-tale ending, a notion that Rishi also seemed to entertain. But his face mirrored the conflict within. She could see that their fairy tale might not unfold as they had envisioned.

When Tanya told him she had done a pregnancy test, he smiled and said, "Oh, so it was negative." She simply shook her head.

She says she'll never forget what she read on his face. It said, "Oh my God, what have we done?"

Rishi hugged her close. While she cried, he assured her that it was going to be okay. Tanya might not get the typical fairy tale, the happily ever after, but she still believed their family would be great. When she left the ship, pregnant with her first child, she was relaxed because she believed they would work. They were going to be together. They were going to have their happy ending.

Initially, Rishi's wife didn't know about Tanya, but when he returned home to Nepal after the contract, he told his wife about everything. Divorce was not an option for them, so although she knew, she didn't want to ever talk about it.

Months later, Tanya's daughter, Mina, was born in Australia in her father's absence. Nevertheless, the announcement of the birth reached Rishi on the ship, marking the start of a new chapter in their unconventional family story. Despite the physical separation, Tanya ensured that the connection between herself and father and daughter thrived through the years with phone calls, messages, and photos. With help from her parents, she and Mina even visited Rishi on his ship, the *Norwegian Gem*.

A few years later, during another visit to the *Norwegian Gem*—coincidently, the same ship on which she had first conceived—Tanya and Rishi conceived their second child. When she found out, she was happy, but the weight of her complicated relationship cast a shadow over what should have been a more joyful experience.

Upon leaving the ship, she visited her parents, who were still living in New York. Watching *The Lion King* on Broadway, Tanya's tears flowed down her face in the darkness. She was silently breaking under the weight of it all.

For the second birth, Tanya and Rishi welcomed another girl, Priya. Tanya was thrilled to have him there this time, and he even took some extended time off the ship for the first few months to be with his Australian family. But it was short lived.

Having and raising their first child by herself had been hard enough, and Tanya was still lonely and struggling with not having the future that she and Rishi had planned. She had been parenting Mina virtually alone for years. The challenges of raising their children on her own wore on her, and she longed for a person to share the joys and tribulations of parenting with. Tanya's yearning for companionship led her to express her desire. She remembers telling Rishi, "I just don't want to be alone anymore. I can't do this alone. I want a partner."

The five years that separated the births of their daughters were challenging, but they underscored the tie Tanya and Rishi had together.

Attempting to keep things uncomplicated, Tanya struggled with her feelings for him, which would not subside, and she told him so. Rishi, in turn, shared his plans to make money and build a house in Nepal with a room for Tanya and their children to live in. She remained skeptical, unsure if this was merely a dream or a genuine commitment to a shared future. The looming presence of his family in Nepal—who, apart from his wife, knew nothing of them—created a barrier that hindered her from envisioning a lasting connection.

The cultural differences between them came to the forefront when Rishi explained the Nepalese belief that staying with someone for a few weeks equates to marriage. He also talked about acceptance in Nepalese culture, where having multiple wives was not uncommon. Tanya, holding on to her Western ideals, found herself unable to both accept these ideals and a future that was so unstable.

The divide posed insurmountable challenges not only for Tanya but for Rishi's family as well. At his wife's request, Rishi signed off ships and returned to Nepal to work in farming, leaving

Tanya alone but connected through daily conversations. With Rishi back in Nepal and supporting his family, the nature of their relationship underwent a transformation. Daily conversations evolved into sporadic exchanges, and the emotional distance grew. Tanya, hurt by the dwindling communication, struggled to relinquish the love that always stayed close, though slightly out of reach.

Rishi attempted to secure visas to see Tanya and the girls in Australia, but that proved to be an emotional marathon. The lengthy process, coupled with the heartrending toll it took on both parties, made them realize that their dreams of a shared life were fading. The practicalities of Rishi supporting his family in Nepal hindered any possibility of a more permanent arrangement.

The internal conflict between her desire for intimacy and the realities of their relationship pushed at Tanya daily. In an attempt to alleviate her loneliness, she and Rishi negotiated to allow her to explore casual physical relationships while remaining committed to him emotionally, but she could not move on. The pain of the separation led Tanya to dark places, manifesting in depression when Rishi was not present. Because his absences were becoming more frequent, their sporadic online interactions became a lifeline, a brief respite from the solitude, only to return to sadness when the screen darkened.

Eventually recognizing the unhealthy nature of their relationship, Tanya came to understand the importance of letting go. Her travels to the ship and Nepal were desperate attempts to bridge the emotional chasm that grew during their time apart. Tanya felt like a hidden secret, a chapter in Rishi's life concealed from the eyes of his family in Nepal. Their relationship weathered two instances of separation lasting two years each, prompting Tanya to make a personal pact not to endure extended periods without intimacy.

In contrast, Rishi's wife, aware of the story, maintained a veil of secrecy. Tanya yearned for a day when her daughters could meet their extended family. They were unaware of the intricacies of their father's family dynamics and remained enthusiastic about connecting with him. Online video chats allowed them to share moments of joy with the father they adored, but his eighteen-year-old daughter and sixteen-year-old son remained blissfully unaware of their sisters in Australia.

Tanya had anticipated a reunion that would never materialize. Acknowledging that prompted her to release the expectations she had held on to for so long and to start creating distance that transcended the physical miles.

Tanya and Rishi spoke every day for several years until their communication slowed. Then they talked once every few months. She was hurt by this, and still had strong feelings for him. But she didn't think their relationship was all for nothing. It had taught her a lot, such as how to be emotionally independent as a woman and how to be alone. For her own mental health and for her daughters, she knew she had to take a step back. Tanya's tale of endurance—tested by time, distance, and cultural differences—is a common one for ships.

When I first met Tanya in 2017, eight years after Tanya and Rishi had first met, he and his wife and family were still living together. The intricate web of unspoken truths surrounding his family not knowing about her and the girls continued to cast a shadow over Tanya's longing for her daughters to meet their extended family in Nepal, who were still concealed in secrecy. It seemed that neither Tanya nor Rishi's wife wanted to lose him.

Tanya's odyssey of emotions and self-discovery made an indelible mark on me. She stood at a crossroads, armed with the wisdom she'd gleaned, And while it was so hard to break away from the dream, she knew it had to be done. Yet she believed that she and Rishi would always be open to picking up where they'd left off. I worried that, due to their unshakable love, she might be unable to move on.

Chatting with Tanya again years later, in 2024, I discovered that my worries had been unfounded. Not only had a lot changed, but coincidentally, when we did our Zoom call, she and her daughters were in Nepal for a visit. I also had the pleasure of meeting Rishi on that call and chatting with him.

Tanya now works as a leather sewing machinist, mainly making guitar straps, and she loves her job. "I'm very good at it, and it makes me happy," she told me. The girls are growing quickly and doing well. Mina is now fifteen and has a job and a boyfriend. Priya is ten and an energetic "chatterbox."

When the goalposts of the times Tanya and Rishi could be together constantly changed, she found herself forever disappointed and, eventually, defeated. But during an *ayahuasca* ceremony—an event in which participants hope to connect with spirits and their inner selves to initiate spiritual healing—she made a breakthrough.

"I thought I was getting over everything, but I wasn't completely over it," she said. "Everything came back to me. Rishi's wife, the guilt, the situation with his family, my daughters in the middle . . . I cried a thousand tears. But it allowed me to work through it, accept what was, and forgive myself and Rishi deeper than I already had."

Tanya said it had been hard to move on from her romantic feelings, but she'd craved physical love and affection, because she is human. To my surprise and delight, she told me she was in a relationship. Frankly, I had been worried that Tanya would still be single and committed to a man who couldn't be with her.

When we spoke, she had been with her partner, Jacky, for three years, and he lived with them. Jacky is a fun and resourceful Frenchman from Réunion, a small island near Madagascar. He had moved to Australia with his previous wife, whom he'd met while travelling through France. Years earlier, he and Tanya had hit it off as friends, but just three years ago, they had reconnected, admitting to always feeling a spark for one another. They had quickly became a couple. Tanya says Jacky's love language is acts of service, and he is very caring. They work together processing leather goods, and they're doing an introductory upholstery course together. Jacky also has two children, of similar ages to Tanya's girls, who live with his wife. The girls are warming up to Jacky.

Rishi admitted that it was very hard when he told Tanya to move on with her life without him, to be happy. When she got together with Jacky, it was clear that this person was very special to her, and it killed Rishi. He even started to break down the communication with Tanya and his daughters, claiming he was giving them space out of respect for her new relationship. He later admitted to me, "I was jealous."

Even though Tanya was disappointed with the lack of communication, she kept it up when she could, going as far as planning this current trip to Nepal. "It's always been important to me that the girls know Rishi," she said. "He's a beautiful, wonderful man."

Rishi is still married and living and working in Nepal. His kids are intelligent and accomplished. His daughter is getting her master's in health-care management, and his son is studying engineering and computer science. Mina often says she would like to meet her sister.

When we spoke in the fall of 2024, Tanya and the girls had still not met any of their Nepalese family. While she would have liked her daughters to know their paternal family, Tanya admitted that they're not welcome. Rishi's wife has never forgiven Rishi and Tanya for their ship relationship. "I don't want to encroach on her world," Tanya said. "I don't want to cause trouble or make her uncomfortable. I'm simply here for the girls to see their father." She acknowledged that things work very differently in Nepal, and she wanted to respect everyone's boundaries.

"Once I'm good with their mother, I know my kids will happily accept their sisters," Rishi said.

So on this visit, when we spoke, Tanya and her daughters were keeping their distance. Tanya wasn't staying in Rishi's town but rather in accommodations an hour away.

Rishi's wife knew that Tanya and her husband's daughters were there in Nepal, and she wasn't happy about it. She didn't return Rishi's daily calls after he left to be with them.

"She could not stop me from coming," he said.

While I was chatting with Tanya, Rishi popped into the call and introduced himself. He was warm, friendly, and forthcoming about his life. I flat-out asked him if he was happily married. "No. But I stay in my marriage because that is what you do. That's what's done here."

Rishi admitted that his wife takes care of him, his parents, and his children and that they generally get along. But in a perfect world, he would be with both families and travel back and forth between both countries. He says if he were in a different culture, one that accepted divorce, he would be living in Australia.

During our chat, Tanya and Rishi talked about meeting some of their family the following week because this was now the opportunity to do so. But they were unsure, and I was not convinced that it would happen. While the girls know of their two siblings, grandparents, aunts, uncles, and cousins, none of them know the girls exist.

A few days after our follow-up call, I got a Facebook message from Tanya: "My girls met their brother today!"

It must have been a big day for tall and gentle Sandesh. At twenty-one, he not only learned that he has two sisters but got to meet them. The meeting was awkward, and he was shocked. He was initially angry with his father but reached out to him the next day to say that he was glad Rishi had told him.

"Priya gave Sandesh a little hug when he left," Tanya said.

I can't help but wonder if my candid and slightly awkward telephone chat with Rishi that day helped him decide to open up and finally be honest with his son.

While some might judge Rishi's decisions, I want to give him credit. Unlike many of the ship dads, he stayed in touch with the mother of his children—even though it was hard for a number of different reasons—and stayed in his marriage.

"In my kids' generation, this is starting to change. They have more freedom from the rules of our culture," Rishi told me. "But for my generation and my parents', there were always rules and boundaries. I didn't get to eat what I wanted to eat. I didn't get to go where I wanted to go."

There is obvious and genuine love between Tanya and Rishi, even if it's become strictly platonic. Knowing their history, Jacky is likely stirring in his leather boots in Australia while they are together in Nepal, which is totally natural.

Anyone with eyes could see that Rishi was still in love with Tanya. With her sitting right there, he told me, "I'll love this one always. I lost the person I'm in love with, but I'm glad she is happy."

While I struggled to get over what had happened, Luiz made it easier each day by helping make ends meet, through financial support and actively engaging in our daily life. He was exceptionally good with our son. I could clearly see how much he loved Gabriel and wanted nothing but the best for him.

Luiz knew he had to build my trust and respect back up and worked at that every day. I watched him mature and act more like himself and not like the cold, cocky guy I had thought he was, the one I met on the ships. He started to open up and be silly and vulnerable, the person he actually was, not the act he had once put on. Moving past "the issue" was a deeply personal journey that involved giving myself time to process my emotions as well as lots of self-care. Luckily, Luiz was ready and willing to give me all the time I needed. Day after day, he stayed consistent, and I found myself becoming happier. As we reconnected and he rebuilt my trust, he went from sleeping in the spare bedroom to slowly migrating back into my bed.

It became clear that Luiz had no intention of going anywhere. He was here to stay—which meant we had to legally secure his residency in Canada. Upon hearing all the stories of the issues you can face with the paperwork, we hired an immigration lawyer—with the little money Luiz had—who advised us against the application we had been working on.

We had been living together for almost a year, so she said our best shot was for me to sponsor Luiz into the country as my common-law partner. To prove that we were, in fact, a couple, we had to gather letters from friends and family, proof of our joint bank account, photographs of us together, screenshots from our texts and messages, and much more. This made the process longer, but the lawyer assured us that it was a stronger application.

During the process, the three of us even had to leave the country and enter again on a wing and a prayer—hoping that Canada Border Services would let Luiz back in to reset his tourist visa. Our cheapest option was a rundown resort in Cuba for a week, which was cheaper than a weekend in France's Saint-Pierre and Miquelon, two small islands that lie just off the coast of Newfoundland.

Our worried families stood by the day we returned, concerned that we wouldn't be let back into Canada. I believe that Gabriel, just one year old, was the perfect cute distraction for the immigration officials. Luckily, it worked out and they let us into Canada with no issue. The relief was palpable; I could feel the stress leave my body.

Things had been rough, and some men would have given up. Not Luiz. He stood his ground, saying that he didn't care what he needed to do. He wanted to be with us and would do whatever it took.

The immigration process, which would take us years and thousands of dollars, was exhausting.

Anyone who says immigrating to Canada is easy has not done it.

Living solely on my maternity-leave benefits, we struggled to pay bills because Luiz wasn't legally allowed to work in Canada. We had no money and were living off of egg sandwiches and noodles. As long as Gabriel had everything he needed, we were okay with eating cheap ramen every night. We knew that being together would be an uphill battle but were absolutely willing to put in the work.

Even in tough times, we seemed to thrive—to everyone's surprise, including ours. Most friends and family assumed we would never last. We'd once had everything going against us, but despite all the ups and downs, we eventually fell in true love. We both had the fervour to nurture and maintain the relationship with communication, compromise, and support. We built our emotional intimacy, which was critical for our strong and resilient relationship. Although learning about the dishonestly on board had been emotionally devastating, I know now that it's possible to recover and ease your pain over time because I did exactly that. Time and patience healed the wounds.

My dream of becoming a mother and having a family had come true, and I felt beyond lucky.

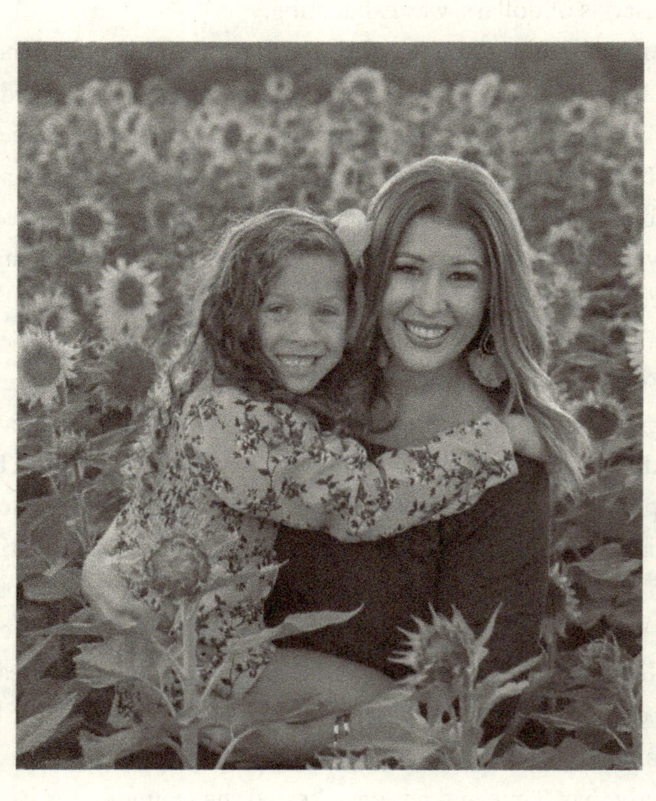

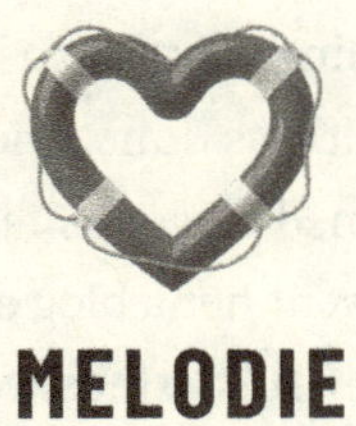

MELODIE

Melodie, a teacher from the United States, had been married for ten years when she finally decided to get a divorce. Her ex-husband had severe mental health problems and was physically and emotionally abusive. Throughout the marriage, he continually tried to get Melodie to try and have a baby. She kept herself busy getting her master's degree, training, and running marathons to avoid the possibility. Because of their domestic problems, she did everything that she could do to put off having kids with him.

Then, two years after they were married, she found out that her husband had a nine-year-old daughter. In fact, not only did Melodie learn he had a daughter, but the daughter was coming to live with them full-time because her mother was an alcoholic and was going to rehab. Suddenly, Melodie was the full-time stepmom of a preteen girl.

She watched and hated how her husband parented his daughter, while at the same time developing a quick bond with the girl.

They leaned on each other and needed each other. They made a pact that Melodie wouldn't leave until she had graduated from high school. When the time came, Melodie took off and asked for nothing. He kept everything apart from her car, dog, and clothes. But it was okay because it was done. She had escaped.

Melodie was determined to get as far away from her former life as possible. A friend sent her a blog entitled *40 Ways to Make Money While You Travel*. Cruise ships were on the list, and jobs working with children—which she was very qualified for, with her education and teaching experience—were offered.

After a whirlwind recruiting process, at the age of thirty-two, Melodie found herself with Royal Caribbean Cruises, working as a member of the youth staff on board. Suddenly, she was in a completely different atmosphere, which was exactly what she needed at the time. Ship life made her feel like she was in college again. Like a lot of "new hires," she kind of went crazy when she joined the ships and partied hard.

She worked on ships for about two years and had the time of her life. During those two years, she worked on four different Royal Caribbean ships, doing five-month contracts on each one. She visited forty-two countries, experienced culture she had only seen on TV, met people with the most vibrant personalities, and laughed more than she had ever laughed in her life.

She joined her fourth ship, *Brilliance of the Seas*, at its port in Harwich, England. After just two weeks on board, Melodie met John. As usual, the pair met at the crew bar. A musician from Nigeria, John had grown up in England. Melodie couldn't get enough of this beautiful bass player with a British accent. Immediately, she was hooked.

They had an odd courtship that conflicted culturally. She was the stereotypical "strong, independent American woman" type, while he had chivalrous Nigerian ways and wanted to be in control. Like those in many ship relationships, they spent most of their time together, but there was never any discussion of monogamy.

Melodie got pregnant within the first two weeks of meeting him even though she was on birth control. One day she started to feel nauseous in the crew mess—which on a good day smells like death—and then suddenly, her usually clear skin was getting pimples. Something was up.

So when the ship was in Maine, she got off, dodging friends to find a Rite Aid Pharmacy and buy a pregnancy test. She took it back to the ship and peed on the stick. Not believing it was possible, she quickly found out she was, in fact, pregnant. To add insult to injury, she had gangway duty in half an hour. She had to smile and welcome people back on the ship when all she wanted to do was cry.

John's reaction to the news was good. "I kinda thought you were." He assured her that everything would be all right.

Melodie, on the other hand, cried for days, knowing she had to tell her family members, who were very much the "you don't have kids out of wedlock" type.

To add to the anxiety of telling her family, Melodie's only sister had recently found out she was pregnant with a baby she'd tried for and really wanted. But then she'd had a miscarriage two days before Melodie found out she was pregnant. Melodie ended up on Skype one day with her sister and realized she needed to know before their parents found out.

Melodie ripped off the Band-Aid and dropped the baby bomb: "So, you're not going to be a mom in May, but you're going to be an aunt in May."

And as Melodie watched her sister react, she heard her mother in the background. "What? Oh, my goodness. Who is that?"

"Um, yeah. So, Mom's here," her sister said.

Mom's initial reaction? Two statements: "Who is the father?" and "At least you won't be drinking as much anymore."

Fortunately, her sister reacted very positively about the baby-to-be. She stepped up and became Melodie's rock, keeping in touch frequently and sending care packages to the ship with books and items for her pregnancy. Melodie wanted the opportunity to tell her dad, but her mom ended up telling him. Her parents were very disappointed and didn't talk to her again for two months.

One random day while Melodie was off the ship at a mall in Maine, her parents called.

"Hello," she said meekly, worried about what was coming next.

"Okay, so we've opened up a storage unit, and we have some friends who have a bunch of furniture they don't want anymore. So when you come home, we'll help out and . . . "

Support and unconditional love from two parents who just needed a minute—or two months—to get it together. In any case, they told Melodie they would be there with her through this entire thing and help with whatever she needed. It was tough for them to accept, but in the background, they hustled to create a safe space for her to come home to. Melodie describes that day as a complete shock but also one of the happiest days of her life.

As time passed on the ship, Melodie, already overcome, grew more stressed. Suddenly the age gap between her and John, who was just twenty-five, was getting more and more noticeable. Melodie acknowledged this and didn't want to take away the "life" of a travelling Nigerian musician by asking him to settle down in Kansas. She didn't really have expectations or romantic fantasies of them being a happy family, but rather envisioned him maybe coming to visit from time to time.

John didn't want to tell any of their fellow crew members about the baby. Melodie told some close friends and co-workers who would inevitably have found out, due to her unusual lack of drinking and her body's changes.

One night the youth staff were out at the crew bar, welcoming a new male co-worker who had just signed on. The crew sat together and welcomed their new team member, pointing out the "who's who" on the back deck.

"Here's where the entertainers sit, there's where the casino crowd sits, that guy there is Melodie's baby daddy, the smoking section is—"

John saw Melodie's co-worker pointing at him, and in a drunken, heated misunderstanding, he pushed the crew member, who ended up hitting his head hard on a wall.

You put hands on someone on a ship? Zero tolerance.

John immediately ran from the party, knowing full well he was about to be detained by on-board security. He would be put into seclusion in preparation for being kicked off at the next port. There was no doubt he would be fired.

Being pregnant, Melodie wasn't out at the bar that night. Rather, she was awakened by a phone call from her co-worker, riled up by the drama after being assaulted.

"You need to find your boyfriend because he just knocked me

out when he pushed me up against the wall. They're looking for him. The security team is trying to find him."

Frantically, she looked for John, eventually finding him sitting in the corner of a barely used crew internet room, drunk and defeated.

"I don't want anybody saying bad stuff about me, about us, and he was pointing at me! It was just to protect you," he blubbered.

Melodie made him get up, and they hurried to her room where, minutes later, security officers knocked on the door. They took him into custody and quarantined him in a room.

Melodie followed them. "I'm pregnant with his child. I need to talk to him. I need to see him."

"Sorry. Not going to happen," they told her. They wouldn't let anybody see him and placed a guard to sit outside his door.

For John's last two days on the ship, Melodie could talk to him on the phone, and that was it. In an attempt to see him before he disembarked, she went to the gangway and waited for the line of signoffs to make their way out. Security officers stood by the door, letting the line go ahead of John. Security on board tried to stay patient, knowing the dynamics.

"I'll be messaging you as soon as I get off the ship, and everything's gonna be okay," John said. "We're gonna make this happen, and it's going to be amazing."

That was the last time Melodie saw John.

Two months later, when she was almost six months pregnant, Melodie signed off the ship and went back home to the US. She and John had been in touch from time to time, but it was complicated. Most conversations led to arguments, so it was easier to just not talk at all.

Melodie admits that when she was first pregnant, in a moment of weakness, she messaged John's sister on Instagram: "Your brother is never going to tell you this, but he's going to have a child." She was mad at him for not wanting to tell anybody—namely his family—his "dirty little secret." John's sister never responded and then blocked her on Instagram.

Melodie was trying to figure out the next steps and took a job as a leasing consultant in an apartment complex. When her due date came, there was still no baby. A few days later, because she was feeling good and preferred to keep working, she volunteered to take someone's shift. That morning, she started early labour. Feeling okay, she worked that full day, went home that night, and went to bed for a few hours—until she was awakened in the morning by contractions. It was a Sunday. Like every Sunday, her family was at church, so she took a shower, carefully put on her makeup, and drove herself to the hospital.

On the drive to the hospital, she messaged back and forth with John, letting him know what was going on. He had been pretty much out of the picture for most of the pregnancy, but all of a sudden, he insisted on helping name the baby. Melodie had already chosen the name Aria for her, but John wanted her name to be Naomi, which means "woman of God." It was just one more point of contention between them, and what with being in active labour, Melodie wasn't interested in an argument.

After about fifteen hours of labour, her doctor decided on a C-section, which took fifteen minutes.

It was love at first sight. Melodie sent John a photo of his daughter, Aria Ann Naomi.

"She's beautiful," he said when he called. Then he uttered a phrase Melodie has become very familiar with over the years: "I can't wait to come and visit her."

Melodie wasn't resentful of him in that moment. Instead, she thanked him for giving her the best gift. He had given her something she never dreamt that she would have wanted.

At the beginning, John and Melodie used Skype from time to time so he could see Aria. But he never helped out financially, and she never pushed it. A couple of times, John said he was going to come visit, but it never panned out.

Once he was in Vegas because his band was playing a gig there, and he called her. "I'm going to come see you and Aria tomorrow. Can you come pick me up at the airport? Flight gets in at eight tomorrow morning, and I can . . ."

Melodie stopped him and told him no. Absolutely not.

"This is not how we do things. If you want to see your daughter, we can plan it on my terms."

She told him to change his ticket destination to Beijing, where he was living at the time, because she wouldn't be at the airport to get him. And that was that.

When I chatted with Melodie in 2019, Aria was almost four years old. John had sent her a couple of Christmas and birthday presents and had reached out every few months. When Aria is older, Melodie says she'll support her if she wants to try and get to know her father better. But for now, she's content to leave things as is.

Melodie isn't sad at all about the way that any of this has gone down. At the beginning, she admits she was caught up in the madness of ship life and used to struggle and fight with John. But now she looks back on it like it was very silly.

John doesn't play a fatherly role in Aria's life, and the girl knows nothing about him. She tells people that she doesn't have a dad. Melodie feels that while her daughter is young and not at an age where she's asking who her father is, why confuse and possibly disappoint her.

When the inevitable day comes, Melodie plans to talk about John in a positive light: "I'll talk about how he's a musician and plays music and lives in other countries and travels the world. Some sort of, like, fantasy person."

Melodie doesn't hold anything against John and wants him to live his life and be happy. She believes that's what he is doing right now, so she's happy for him. He's got an amazing kid, and if he ever wants to get to know her, it can be arranged. But on Melodie's terms.

Melodie watches her friends who must share custody and feels great about her set-up. She and her daughter share an incredible bond and are so happy and content.

Months before our interview, Melodie took Aria for her first cruise. As soon as they stepped onto the ship, Aria came alive. Every time she heard music or saw a stage or an opportunity to have an audience, she entertained folks by dancing and just being generally adorable. Days into the cruise, the whole ship knew her: crew and passengers.

When Melodie had worked on board, one of her favorite things to do had been to sit on the back deck and watch the ship sail away from shore. After the Sailaway Party, where Aria killed it with her dance moves, Melodie took her daughter to the back of the ship to watch the sailaway. She said it had been an incredibly peaceful moment in time.

She had cried and taken photos of her excited first-time cruiser. "I thought, my life has come full circle right now. Sitting on the back of a cruise ship with my little cruise-ship baby in such a different, but wonderful, place."

When I caught up with Melodie again in 2024, a lot had changed. She had always been a beautiful, stylish woman. However, I couldn't help but notice that she looked even better than the last time I had seen her. In fact, she was glowing, and I told her as much. I soon learned it was the glow of love. She had met her partner after an unfortunate string of terrible dates. She had noticed him on her dating app because he'd posted photos of water skiing, something she also loves, and reached out. They hit it off immediately and have been together for almost three and a half years.

The cherry on top is that they have kids of the same age who get along well. And even more importantly, her partner is fantastic with Aria and loves her so much. He's become an incredible male role model in her life.

"I don't know how I got so lucky to be living this life right now," Melodie said.

John has still not met Aria. As far as we know, his religious Nigerian parents and extended family still don't know about her. They would very likely disapprove of him getting someone pregnant out of wedlock and then not marrying the mother or supporting the child. And they would probably be most upset about all the time that Aria and John have missed. He lives between Spain and London, still performs in bands, and lives that music-industry lifestyle. He checks in with Melodie about once a month, and she sends him photos and videos. If she's done something exciting that Melodie thinks he would like to see, such as the first day of school or a gymnastics competition, she sends him something.

John responds that their daughter is amazing and beautiful. It seems like the more he sees of her, the more he realizes he is missing out. He has mentioned a few times recently that he would like to travel to the US to meet his daughter, which Melodie would entertain, but she's still unsure of how she feels about that. There would have to be strict, predetermined boundaries if a visit were to happen. For example, Melodie would not let John stay at their home. He would have to stay in a hotel and meet them slowly, in a public place for a few hours, and then build from there.

Aria is now eight years old and the happiest little girl. Almost every day, she says, "Mommy, today was my best day ever!" There is no denying that she looks like her father and has his smile. She also has many of his mannerisms, proving that biology is powerful. Melodie admits that, someday, Aria may want to know about her paternal family, and she doesn't know what that will look like.

So far, Aria hasn't started asking questions.

"You can tell that Aria isn't white, but she doesn't seem to notice," Melodie said. "She doesn't ask why she's darker than Mommy or why her hair is so curly." Melodie said she will likely consult with therapists on the best ways to navigate those questions, as they will inevitably come soon. Melodie wants to ensure the least amount of trauma possible for her daughter. She thinks that the fact John lives so far away will help soften the blow.

Aria has an amazing family that adores her. Melodie's boyfriend's parents—her "bonus grandparents," whom she calls Grammy and Poppa—love the little girl and treat her like part of the family. Melodie's parents, Poppy and Meema, while initially disappointed in their daughter, now often remark that Aria is the best thing that has happened to Melodie and to their family. She's a blessing.

Before we knew it, two years had passed since Luiz's arrival, and his Canadian Permanent Residence application was approved. Exhausted from the mountains of paperwork and the financial struggle, we felt like we had been put through the wringer. It was a great day, and we felt a huge weight lift from our shoulders. We were so thankful when the process was finally completed.

In spring 2019, with generous help from Luiz's family, we travelled to Brazil, to his home city of Petrópolis, Rio de Janeiro, just before Gabriel's second birthday. At that point, Luiz had not seen his family for over four years. I was excited but scared to travel all that way with my most precious cargo. I also felt nervous that they would look at me like an old woman who had taken advantage of their innocent son.

With shaky legs, I walked into the terminal to meet his parents. As soon as I met them, all that fear vanished. After Luiz's mother held her grandson for the first time, she hugged me tightly and repeated the words "thank you" over and over in English. I started to cry, and she did too. We stood holding each other, sobbing. Strangers in the airport watched and couldn't help but tear up at the powerful moment they were witnessing.

The entire family gave Gabriel and me the warmest welcome and were kind and friendly. Gabriel immediately took a special liking to Luiz's father, who is very reserved and shy. He beamed, saying that his grandson wanted to spend more time with him than with anyone else. While there, I often sat in awe, watching Gabriel with his beautiful Brazilian family. I felt an immediate connection to them all, especially Luiz's mother, Paula. Two weeks later, I cried just as much saying goodbye as I had when I met her.

Once back home in Newfoundland, working on gathering the stories of ship moms became a project that kept me motivated while I was starting to have a hard time with other areas of my life.

Our sweet boy was a handful, and parenting wasn't easy. As a toddler, Gabriel often acted without thinking, interrupting others. He was easily frustrated and moody and was taking unsafe risks. We just figured that was standard toddler stuff.

As time passed, though, it got harder, not easier, as conventional parenting tactics seemed not to work on our boy. We knew something was off when he was removed from his first preschool for his behaviour.

It was heartbreaking to watch Gabriel struggle so much. I felt completely overwhelmed by it all, wanting to help him. But I had no idea how.

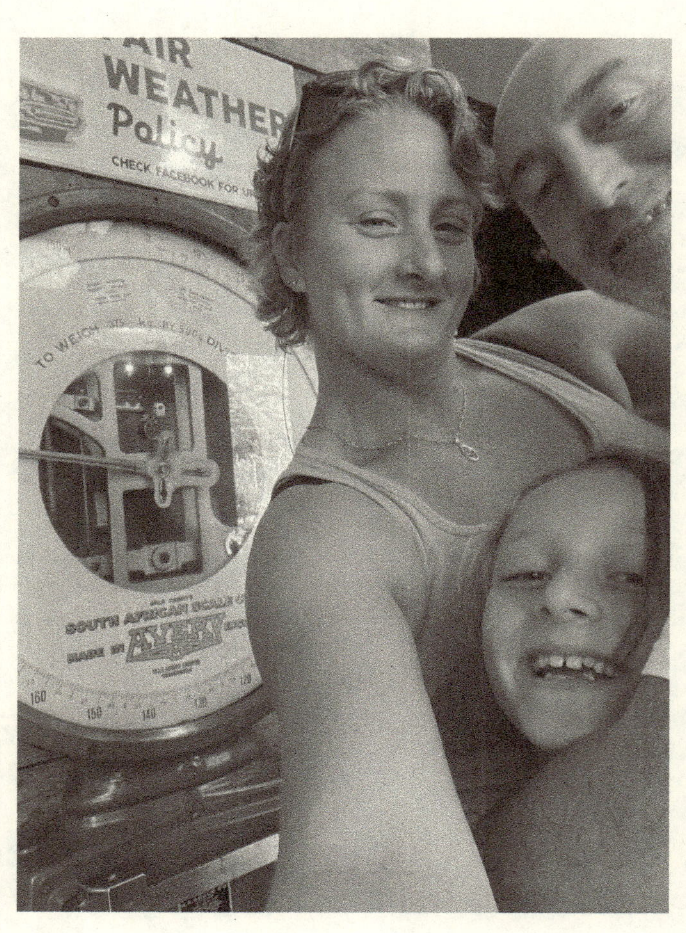
AIR
WEATHER
Policy
CHECK FACEBOOK FOR
TO WEIGH
SOUTH AFRICAN SCALE
MADE IN
AVERY
160
150
140
130
120

SAGE

From the Western Cape of South Africa, Sage started as a personal trainer on the high seas but admitted that she jumped from job to job a lot, getting bored quickly. After working with the Boswell Wilkie Circus, a popular entertainment business in South Africa, she wanted to do something different, to travel even more and see the world. Sage was told about Steiner International, one of the most prominent recruiting agencies for spas, salons, and gyms in the world cruising industry. She applied for work as a personal trainer and, not long after, got hired to work with Celebrity Cruises.

After Sage adjusted, she really enjoyed ship life. She was the type of crew member who fit in so well that she crafted her life at sea for many years: five with Celebrity Cruises and two with Princess Cruises. She knew ship life like the back of her hand, having worked in many different departments—as activities staff, for example—and eventually in administrative roles such as activities manager and purser.

Ship life, often depicted as scandalous, worked for her, but when it came to relationships, she was very tame in comparison to her crew mates. Life aboard the ship was a swirl of parties, camaraderie, and the buzz of rumours that surrounded crew hookups.

Shyer than most on board, Sage acknowledged the truth in those rumours, saying, “Everything is okay—as long as everyone’s in agreement with it, of course.”

Eventually, her ship life took an unexpected turn when she met a quiet Italian engineer, Ciro, whom she immediately found herself crushing on. Sage chuckled as she recalled their first encounters, saying, “He was a lot older than me.” Like Sage, he was more the shy type. But unlike many crew, he was looking for a real relationship.

Ciro really liked Sage but was too nervous to talk to her, so for a while, he admired her from afar. Awkwardly hoping to take their relationship to the next level, he put himself out there and resorted to something he would never usually do. He sent her flowers through an on-board Filipino florist friend. She was very touched by the gift, and while she wasn’t sure who it was from, she had her suspicions. She thought about the engineer but assumed he was married, like all the other on-board engineers.

Not that that mattered to most on board, but it did matter to Sage.

Two weeks later, when she saw Ciro having a drink by himself at the crew bar, she approached him and started talking. After a beer, he finally revealed that he’d sent the flowers. Blushing, he admitted he was intimidated by her and didn’t know how else to approach her. She was flattered, and he was so kind and sweet—and, amazingly, not married!

Slowly—particularly in ship-life terms—they started dating on board. They adored one another and became exclusive. They were both surprised to find that the relationship was easy. Ciro proudly introduced her to his mom over a video call one day, even though she doesn't speak English. A conservative and thoughtful man, he knew he wanted Sage in his life forever.

As the months passed and their connection deepened, he and Sage started joking about having a family. The jokes turned into actual conversations, and before they knew it, they were planning that future and actively trying to get pregnant. They figured they'd wait until they were both on vacation to conceive, but as fate would have it, that was not in the cards. On their first try, they got pregnant.

"Our baby was conceived on the *Caribbean Princess* in Grand Cayman," Sage revealed with a smile.

When the doctor's scan discovered she was, in fact, pregnant, she was happy but nervous because it had happened so quickly, within months. Her partner cried and held her. Ciro couldn't contain his happiness and begged her to let him tell everyone. He was a planner and had everything ready for this major milestone.

After many weeks, Sage finally allowed him to announce the joyous news, and then awaited her departure from ship life. They soon got married in his hometown, on the beautiful and tiny island of Procida, off the coast of southern Italy. The island is mostly Catholic and Sage is not, so the couple's decision to get married not in a church but by a Justice of the Peace was—and remains—the talk of the town. Her family couldn't be there, but they were very much in support of the union.

When the prospect of expanding their family arose, decisions about where to bring their child into the world became paramount. After a lot of thought, the couple decided not to have the baby in South Africa. Italy became their chosen destination, not only because Ciro had a home there, in his hometown that he kept with his aunt, but also because of its European hospital facilities and the coveted Italian passport their child would obtain.

Midpregnancy, Sage packed her bags and made her way to Italy, ready to settle in for a while and prepare to have the baby. When Ciro was done with his following contract, he joined her there. His parents, thrilled to soon meet their grandchild, were very supportive.

Sage didn't speak Italian but was studying it. Ciro's small rural community spoke a very heavy dialect, so while she understood some things, she did struggle daily to understand what people were saying. Being pregnant in a country where she didn't speak the language, she navigated the medical procedures and hospital visits with a mix of determination and helplessness. She struggled to try to describe how her body felt and what she needed at doctor's appointments but remained positive and optimistic about the birth.

It was unfortunate, under those circumstances, that Sage ended up with a complicated delivery. They had planned for a water birth, but after the baby's head got stuck, they unexpectedly transitioned into an emergency C-section. Unlike most, she didn't speak the language of the caregivers, so it became a traumatic experience that she'll never forget. Her husband wasn't even allowed in the operating room. In this sterile environment, communication was a maze of broken English, leaving Sage in a state of exhaustion and vulnerability. Yet, amid the challenges, the medical staff showed kindness and empathy, emphasizing the universal language of care.

A healthy baby boy they called Orion was born, and Sage and Ciro could not have been happier.

With the birth of their son in Italy, Sage embarked on a new chapter of motherhood. When the baby was eight weeks old, she took him to South Africa to meet his family. There, she faced unexpected hurdles while trying to get through immigration. The bureaucratic challenges—to reunite with her family—became a saga of flights, paperwork, and visas. When she and her son made it inside her home country, her family greeted the new addition in tears. There, she received dual citizenship for her boy, who is now officially an Italian South African. The nightmare of a process took an entire year, but Sage is happy she did it.

Because Ciro was working on board, Sage ultimately decided that she and Orion would live in South Africa and not in Procida. This decision was motivated by the desire for a better quality of life for their family. The cost of living was lower, and Orion would have lots of space to play, a bigger home, and lots of activities—not to mention that Sage could be supported by her family, mainly while Ciro was back on ships.

When we spoke in 2019, Orion was four years old. I couldn't wait to hear how the family was when we connected again in 2024. Sage and I caught up about how the past years had been and how the family was doing. Orion, now nine, was a sweet and talented boy with a love for the arts. However, since the last time we'd spoken, they'd discovered something about him.

When Orion started grade school, the administration informed Sage that they suspected he might have ADHD and immediately jumped into gear, offering him services that could help him have successful days in school. Luckily, he was attending a Montessori school, which uses an educational method that builds on children's natural interests and activities rather than formal teaching methods that place an emphasis on hands-on learning.

"We always suspected something different about our boy but couldn't quite put our finger on it," Sage said. "It was never that big of a deal. We just handled the day-to-day incidents in stride."

She admits that sometimes access to these accommodations can be classist, but her family is in a position of privilege to be able to get them.

She also shared that, in the years since we had last spoken, she had also been diagnosed with ADHD and with autism. Neurodiversity, of course, was very familiar to me.

Orion's name means "heaven's light," a shining star pulled right out of the sky. He's now on medication for his ADHD and, with the diagnosis, is able to get extra help and accommodations, which make his life a little easier. He is doing well in school and sprouting up. Recently, he was the lead in a theatre production at their local playhouse, and he killed it, surprising nobody. A shining star.

"Our family is pretty open," Sage said. "We have never been the type of people who need things to be a specific way. The way we approach Orion has changed. He isn't being naughty per se. He may just be sensory overwhelmed or hyperfocused on something."

Sage was extremely forthcoming about how eye-opening the diagnosis had been for both herself and her son. She told me she had done a ton of research about neurodiversity and regrets that she was diagnosed at a later age.

"When I look back at my whole life, I can clearly see it there. My mother and I talked and laughed about how things now made sense," she told me. "I didn't realize I was struggling until I started medication. Soon studying became easier . . . everything became easier!"

Sage says she often felt like she was always behind, trying to catch up with everyone else, but now she has furthered her skills to know how to "take the bull by the horns."

After we had chatted more, I let her know that Gabriel, too, had a confirmed ADHD diagnosis. And though I had yet to officially confirm everything, Sage and I talked about our ongoing work trying to understand both our diagnoses.

These days, she is studying to get her bachelor's degree in health science, majoring in psychology. She'll finish next year but let me know that she plans to continue studying and would like to continue into neuropsychology, which is close to home for her. Her husband, Ciro, still works at sea and is gone quite often, making Sage feel like she's a single mom at times. He plans to retire from ships and has nine years remaining.

When she reflects on the highs and lows of her journey that started on the seas, ventured into Italy, and ultimately settled in the Western Cape of South Africa, she's content. She has embraced her neurodiverse motherhood, leaving ships entirely and becoming a stay-at-home mom going to school for the time being.

Sage has decided that one child is enough, given the demands of Ciro's maritime lifestyle. A long-distance relationship can be challenging at times, but Sage emphasizes the importance of staying in constant contact and trying to bridge the physical gap. Ciro is an exception to the rule of ship dads—still with the mother of his child and in the child's life. He adores his wife and son and their unconventional life.

It was impossible for me not to touch on the parallels between Orion and my son, Gabriel. As with Orion, we suspected early on that there was something different with Gabriel. Also, like Orion, when Gabriel started school, the trouble ramped up. The teachers told us that they, too, suspected something and that we needed to talk to our doctor. Unfortunately, like many people in Newfoundland and Labrador, we didn't have access to a family doctor, so this was not a simple request.

At the end of the grade-one school year, an administrator called and told me, in a raised voice, "You have to do more. I know you don't have a doctor, but other parents are showing up at walk-in clinics to get what they need. You must do more." This call was like a dagger to my heart.

Luiz and I both worked in non-profits, me in the arts and him in immigration. We didn't make a lot of money but were fulfilled in our jobs. Soon, however, we found ourselves exhausted and overwhelmed. To be told I needed to do more about Gabriel's behaviour was rough, but I took the comments to heart, and I did more. I took a week off work and spent every day that week showing up at walk-in clinics, knocking on doors, and calling every medical professional who was listed.

When I got nowhere, Gabriel and I started showing up in the emergency room. The staff would tell me, "We can't help you," and I would say, "Okay, but just so you know, I'm coming back tomorrow." Of course, this wasn't an emergency, but I was determined to be the squeakiest wheel our health district had ever witnessed.

By the end of the week, I got a phone call and was told Gabriel had a doctor. I was also told that this was not a result of my incessant showing up and calling, but I'm sure it didn't hurt. We arrived at his first appointment prepped with so much paperwork and so many details that he was diagnosed with ADHD right away. He was eventually put on medication, but the challenges didn't disappear. Things got worse before they got better.

Our poor boy cycled through medications that made his skin crawl and turned him into a different person. At the peak of the worst trouble, he was having full-on, explosive breakdowns nightly, during which he damaged our home and hit us and himself.

I admit I was constantly overwhelmed by Gabriel, so much so that sometimes, I would lash out and raise my voice. I screamed at him. I started to develop a lot of anger, and I was letting both of our disorders take control of me. Then I came to the sad realization that the parenting I was doing—the only parenting I knew—was the worst kind for him. I had to take a dramatic turn. Normal rule making, household routines, and consequences were simply not working. If I wanted Gabriel to succeed, there were also changes that I needed to make.

This took time and patience, and even as I write these words, I know I'm still not exactly where I want to be in my understanding of how to best parent my special little boy. But I am learning more every day. While it's heartbreaking that he knows he has been labelled as a disobedient child and friends are hard to come by, I am finally—after years—seeing some good progress.

Parenting an ADHD child can be exhausting. Your day might be filled with tantrums, looking for things your child "lost," dealing with careless mistakes, and redirecting. Sage's ability to see her son through his hard times inspired me. "I think the most significant thing that has helped me is letting go of how I thought it should be," she told me.

Sage's parenting methods were well researched and thought out, and her boy succeeded. I was still waking up more and more worried every day. Gabriel was having a difficult time with daycare and school, with issues being reported almost daily. We did start to get access to the programs and services we needed to help Gabriel have more successful days at school. That was helpful but not really cutting it.

My already-short fuse was shortening more and more each day. Acknowledging that I was feeling overwhelmed, I started therapy, which made me look at my neurodevelopmental disorders. It was becoming clear that I had likely passed these down to my son. I became depressed, angry, and anxious. Soon the therapist told me I might benefit from antidepressants. I had never taken them before and welcomed the help. I immediately noticed the bottle had a little sticker on it: "Do not drink alcohol while taking this medicine."

I was still drinking from time to time, bingeing when I did but trying to limit the drinks. But as one can expect, as soon as the drinks produced the buzz, I felt stimulated and uninhibited and would start throwing back more drinks, chasing the buzz. Soon enough, I went from blacking out once every ten or so times that I drank to blacking out every second time. I would not only black out at night but would also suffer so badly during the day or two following that I couldn't parent, work, or be a contributing partner. Drinking started taking up a lot of space in my life. Every time I drank, two to three days would go to recovering, and—soon enough—I started saying out loud, for the first time, "I think I need to stop drinking."

The truth is, I can't drink like a normal person. I never could. I'm not an alcoholic in the way most people think of it. I could always go months and not drink. My issue has always been that, when I start drinking, I cannot stop. Like a lot of my fellow Newfoundland and Labradorians, I'm a binge drinker. Drinking heavily is very normal in this place, if not somewhat celebrated.

When the buzz of alcohol hits me, it doesn't matter if I have work the next day or have no money in the bank. I'm so impacted by the buzz that I then binge. A lot of people would say this makes no sense, that your next drink is a choice. Just stop at two drinks. It's not hard! But that's just it. It's not just hard but almost impossible for me to stop. A therapist once told me that I have a drug- and alcohol-usage disorder, and that sounds right to me. I can have the first drink but the second drink—and every one after that—has me.

But I thought I had my drinking under control. I thought that the one out of ten times that I blacked out wasn't a big deal and that the social and fun benefits well outweighed those times. Some of the funnest times in my life have been over drinks. My blackouts, while scary for me, weren't visible to anyone, because I seemed fine to friends. The lights were on, but nobody was home.

I have blacked out then made out with people who, the next day, were upset when they realized I didn't remember anything. In some cases, I had no regrets—but wished I'd been in the world so I could remember! In other cases, I carried trauma over not knowing exactly what had happened, and those blackouts played on my mind. Some of these incidents happened with friends who genuinely didn't know how intoxicated I was, because I was walking around talking to people like normal, albeit overly happy. I seemed coherent.

But other incidents happened while I was very obviously intoxicated. For example, someone grabbing the hair on my head, pulling me over from a garbage bucket—with my face and mouth still covered in vomit—and putting my head onto their crotch. There has been more than one circumstance that I didn't want to be in, starting as young as my teenage years. While I don't mean to generalize, all my traumatizing blackout experiences have been with men. The experiences were often with acquaintances, but sometimes they were with "friends."

My second-last time drinking, I threw up all over a cab and then spent the next day trying to find the driver, to thank them and give them a tip for getting me home covered in barf, but safely.

The last time I drank alcohol was New Year's Eve, December 31, 2023. I drank fancy gin cocktails made at home by Luiz, who utilized his former bartending skills to create drinks in my favourite flavours, Earl Grey and citrus. Luiz and I drank and rang in a quiet New Year with just one other couple, bestie friends Ginnie and Chandra, having no idea or intention that this would be my last time drunk.

All was well until shortly after midnight, when everything went black. When the blackout came, I knew the spins would come shortly after. I puked all over the bathroom. Knowing I had house guests for the night, I drunkenly cleaned it up as I went, thinking I'd done a great job.

The next morning, I woke feeling like death warmed over, not remembering the night before and going into the bathroom to discover that my cleaning job was awful and the bathroom had specks of vomit everywhere. I started throwing up again, but this time it didn't stop for hours. I would drink water and, minutes later, would throw it up. If I didn't drink water, my body would jolt and heave with nothing coming out. Soon I started throwing up a bright yellow, acidic substance, stomach bile, which burned when it came up. I forced water in, trying to throw up anything but the bile. For a long time, I continued to switch from being asleep on the bathroom floor to having my head in the toilet.

After taking a long, glorious drink of water that seemed to be staying down, I fell asleep on the floor for some time. Then I woke with a shudder and felt like I was about to throw up my dinner from last week. I popped up on my two feet, crouched down with my head in the toilet, and let it rip. The heaving was so powerful that I felt my insides let go, and I peed all down my legs into my slippers. But I didn't move because the vomit was still coming.

When it finally let up, I lay on the floor next to my urine puddle until I found the strength to move and clean it up. While I was on my knees cleaning the mess, something inside didn't feel right—like something inside me hadn't been there before. I started to panic, trying to remember if I'd taken out my tampon from the previous night. I didn't find a string so assumed I had, but I had been blackout drunk.

After help from my loving partner, Luiz, I got on the phone for guidance from my licensed practical nurse friend, Chandra—the same one I'd been drinking with the night before. We discovered that it wasn't a tampon I was feeling. I had thrown up so powerfully, heaved so forcefully, that I had expelled my IUD.

The doctor told me it was a perfect storm situation, one that very rarely happens. The combination of my crouching, being on my period, and my insides heaving so intensely resulted in pushing out my contraceptive device.

As many women know, getting an IUD is no walk in the park. They say, "Some people experience cramping similar to or sometimes more intense than menstrual cramps." Well, in my experience, this was the understatement of the century. The procedure to insert my IUD had been agonizing, and excruciating pain had messed with my body and head for days. I wanted to complain and scream, "False advertising!" to the doctors who tell women it's a regular procedure with little to no pain. (Doctors really need to do better when it comes to women's medical procedures.)

When my doctor asked me if I wanted her to put it back in, I told her I needed some time. I was slightly freaked out about the procedure and by what had just happened.

So there I was, IUD-less and wondering how I could have let myself get so inebriated that I would get so sick I would expel everything, including my own birth control. This was rock-bottom. The good thing about rock bottom is that there's nowhere to go but up.

That day, I knew I was done. Rock bottom would become the foundation on which I would rebuild a new life without alcohol. The fun of drinking was no longer outweighing the cons. This wasn't a planned New Year's resolution, but rather an out-of-the-blue realization of a commitment that I needed to make not only for myself but also for my family, to be my best self for them.

My sisters all joke that I am the poster child for learning things the hard way, and I have tons of examples of this. I was reminded again when, seven weeks later, feeling nauseous, rundown and bloated, the reality hit me. I went to the drugstore. Back home, for just the second time in my life, I peed on the stick. The two pink lines took no time to appear. I was shocked. I had gone my whole life having unprotected sex and even, at one point, had actively tried to get pregnant for an entire year. I had never once had a scare.

Here I was, a forty-three-year-old woman who had just pushed out her own IUD, and two months later, I was pregnant again. I figured either Luiz has "supersperm," or we're so biologically compatible that we could get pregnant by lying next to each other. There was no way I could put my body through pregnancy again, especially at this age.

Whatever the reason, one thing was certain. Both Luiz and I were irrefutably on the same page: one and done.

ALL THE OTHER SHIP MOMS

With almost one hundred submissions received, I wish I could have interviewed every ship mom personally because so much story is hidden between the lines.

At the end of each interview, I would tell my ship mom that I had some stats from a survey I wanted to share to see how they felt about the results.

My survey was entirely unscientific, based on just the limited number of women I could reach. This is a very small number in comparison to the actual number of cruise-ship crews. For my stats to represent the reality of those crews, I should have had many more mothers and fathers from the Philippines, India, and Indonesia. And it's probably not just a coincidence that many of the moms selected for this book were from the Royal Caribbean crew, as I was with Royal and involved with the Royal Moms Facebook page.

Of the respondents, the highest percentage of ship moms came from South Africa and Peru, with the Philippines and

Canada not far behind. The rest came from a wide range of countries in the global north and south.

Ship dads also came from disparate countries around the globe, with India and the Philippines being the most common—which lines up with general crew-nationality statistics—followed by England, Croatia, and the United States.

As imperfect as these statistics are, they do paint an interesting picture.

Thirty-seven percent of the ship moms are still with the father of their ship baby.

Nineteen percent of ship moms are in contact with the father but don't have a relationship with them.

Forty-three percent of these sweet mixed-nationality babies, sadly, have no contact with their fathers.

Thirty-five percent of the babies have met or know their father's family.

Thirty-four percent of the babies have not met their father's family.

Thirty-one percent of respondents said the father's family doesn't know about the child.

These statistics are a great reminder of how lucky Gabriel and I are to have Luiz and his family. While I was prepared to become a single mom with no support, I am so grateful not only to have a great coparent, but one I am in love with.

As I documented these ship moms' stories, a common thread emerged. These women all had invaluable lessons to teach me about the true meaning of family, the importance of connection, and how to navigate the unpredictability of life.

Some broke my heart, and others repaired it. Through the

project, a little support network took shape. It became a lifeline for me, someone who had once felt isolated and unintentionally started writing a book. I was lucky to receive so many responses to my call for ship moms that I couldn't interview everyone who shared their story. But all were special, and I was thankful and joyous when reading every single one.

Many of the moms talked about what it was like to have a child with a mixed nationality. So many lovely stories of mixed nationalities came together and worked to create a wonderful multicultural life for their children. As communication technology improves, mixed-nationality or mixed-race couples and families will undoubtedly become more common. It's a unique growing experience for these families, but it doesn't come without its share of issues.

Blended families are often asked, "Where are you from?" This question is complex for a person of mixed nationality or race. It messes with their sense of belonging. Everyone growing up thinks their family structure is "normal" because it's all they know. But outside, extended family, friends, and strangers often make overt comments and commit microaggressions, even unintentionally. The family structure might focus on one culture over another, which can be confusing and backfire. It can lead to shame of one's culture and not pride.

"We have very different cultural backgrounds, but our differences make us stronger," said one Danish ship mom.

One English ship mom was proud of her son's multicultural life saying, "Made in China. Discovered in South Korea. Confirmed in Singapore. Manufactured in England. Born in the United States."

Patience and respect are paramount in blending multiple cultures. While some families blend seamlessly, one parent might actively embrace their partner's culture, while another might struggle to accept and understand their partner. If children are lied to about their heritage, it can lead to confusion and resentment. Kids should be exposed to both cultures and, in turn, to all cultures. Parents can then trust their children to navigate and identify as they see fit for themselves as they grow.

So to that end, people, mind your own business. You are not entitled to know the origins of a stranger. Families and children come in all different types of ways. They are all valid.

While some families come together unexpectedly, others come to be in confusing and upsetting ways. Rape and sexual assault are the most common crimes committed on cruise ships,[1] and even then, many go unreported by victims—specifically, by crew members who have been assaulted by other crew members. The reasons people don't report their assaults vary. Many want to avoid being victimized for a second time and avoid any retaliation. Remember, a cruise ship makes for close quarters. Sometimes, power dynamics come into play, and people—primarily women but also men—are taken advantage of by those in positions of authority.

One Chinese ship mom shared her story with me, but admittedly, I wasn't shocked by the sad story of how she was raped while working on board.

This woman and her roommate were given countless free drinks on the back deck by a fellow crew member, someone they thought was a friend. They both got overly intoxicated, which didn't take much as they were both lightweights. They invited the man back to their cabin to continue drinking. After some time, her friend passed out.

"He wants to have sex. I don't want sex and say no, but he makes me," she told me.

She was then raped while her friend drunkenly snored in the bunk above them. Her assailant was a manager on board and a long-time crew member. She was a new hire and in housekeeping. She didn't report the crime. She was unsure if it was a crime. She said she felt responsible because she drank too much alcohol and invited the man to her cabin. She buried down the trauma, finished her contract, and returned to rural China for her three-month vacation. She felt run down and not herself, which she thought resulted from the incident that played on her mind daily. Then she started getting morning sickness. She soon found out she was nine weeks pregnant. Her family was furious, but she didn't tell them the pregnancy was the result of rape. She felt too ashamed. While abortions are generally accessible and accepted nationwide, her family had always been pro-life, and they insisted that she have the baby anyway. They told her that she needed to take responsibility for her choices.

Her daughter is now five years old, and mom loves her daughter more than anything. She is sweet and silly, and the entire family adores her. The father has no idea that he has a Chinese daughter.

If by some chance this Chinese ship mom reads this book—or another ship mom who had a similar experience reads this—please know that this is not your fault. You were not responsible for what happened to you. Sexual assault and rape aren't always violent incidents in dark alleyways where weapons and fighting back are involved. Most often, it happens with someone you know, in a place you once felt comfortable. Sadly, sometimes it happens with someone you once trusted.

I should mention that assault and rape are also a common occurrence among the passengers. The booze flows, and people feel inconspicuous far from home, both on board and while in ports.

Like a small floating city, a cruise ship is filled with many different types of people. Just like any town, there are great people, but there are always some bad people. Just because you are on vacation, don't let your guard down. Put it up a little more. Even if you meet a fellow passenger or crew member and hit it off with them, remember they're still a stranger that you just met, and use caution in how much you share with them. Some of the most charming people sometimes turn into snakes.

Just like on land, I highly recommend that passengers be aware of date-rape drugs. Watch your drink and only drink unopened beverages or those you have watched being prepared. Watch your drinking in general, period. Don't get too drunk. Be vigilant, use the buddy system with fellow travellers, and stay aware of your surroundings. Never let your key card out of your sight, and always check your room when you enter.

Trust can be hard to come by on board, and while crew are encouraged to keep their guard up, many of the crew struggle at the best of times. One of the biggest struggles with trust I have seen is with on-board couples believing their partner is staying faithful to them, mainly if they're not on board together.

One particular story of a South African mom, whom I will call Violet, was eye-opening. I interviewed this mom and her husband and wrote an entire chapter that was dedicated to her. Once the publishing deal was secured, though, she never responded to my emails or social media messages. Maybe she was worried about how she was portrayed. I'll never know.

As with all my ship moms in the book, their approval was of the utmost importance to me, so I have changed her name. I hope she'll read this one day and it will be helpful for her. I wanted her to know the secret I was waiting to tell her in our follow-up interview. Knowing exactly how she felt, I wanted her to know there was no judgment from my end but only empathy.

Ironically, Violet, born and raised in South Africa, signed her first contract on board, the same ship on which my son was conceived, the same one Luiz and I worked on together. Not long after being on board, she met a man I will call Ajay. Like many ship relationships, it got intense quickly, and they fell madly in love. They hoped to get registered as a couple on board and to work and travel together, but they both knew it would be an uphill battle.

Recognizing the challenges of securing another contract that allowed them to stay together, the couple took a decisive step and decided to get married. A few days later, they bought rings in Nassau. The next day, their managers gave them the afternoon off, and they tied the knot in Key West—just the two of them in their matching white shirts and jeans. They had lunch and then went back to work, quickly getting officially registered as a couple. Just two weeks later, Violet became pregnant.

Everything quickly changed, and Violet had to return to South Africa to have the baby and get settled. Ajay had to continue to work on board to support his family, and while he did visit Violet and meet his new daughter, his imminent departure was looming. This would be their life. Violet admitted that, every time he left, it got more complicated. She knew better than anyone what it was like on board.

Violet started to worry about some beautiful ladies also falling for Ajay's smile and "luring him" into their beds. So, as she explained to me, she wanted to know where Ajay was at all times while on board.

"He needs to call me every hour and a half, even if he's sleeping. He has alarms on his phone. I trust him one hundred percent, but I know how ship life is."

I chuckled, thinking this was an exaggeration, but quickly learned it was, in fact, no joke. She said she wanted to know he was "safe," and Ajay agreed to the terms. He admitted the phone and internet would be costly but was willing to oblige. He set an alarm on his phone to remind him to call every hour and a half, twenty-four hours daily. If he was sleeping, he woke up and called. He told me his roommate asked him, "Why are you calling your wife all hours of the night, every hour? Does she not trust you?"

Once, when he didn't call, Violet went on his Facebook Messenger and messaged a guy she knew of on board. She said, "I know you're on *Rhapsody*. I'm Ajay's wife. Can you call his room and tell him to call me?" And he did.

As I mentioned, this story and ship mom were very special to me. When Violet's face appeared on the Skype screen, my guilty conscience made me twitch a little. She was just as pretty as her photos on Facebook. The truth was, I was keeping a secret. I already knew Violet. I had looked at pictures of her well before

I ever conceived this ship-moms project. When Luiz was on ships living his best life, he added pretty ladies from all over the world to Facebook. I was at home being a single mom, post-partum, with my self-esteem in the toilet. And Violet was one of the "gorgeous, perfect, young girls" I embarrassingly admitted to creeping years previously.

I couldn't wait to tell her, to see her response. But after I chatted with her and her husband, I knew I wanted to wait. Her worry seemed too fresh and too raw at the time.

The way Violet talked about her relationship and the request for Ajay's constant check-ins made me think about all the reasons why she wanted these points of contact and about how she was probably feeling precisely like I felt when I was creeping her on Facebook. From the get-go, I knew I wanted to tell her about my online stalking story, like, "Ha, ha, how about that!" to get her reaction, but I never got the opportunity.

If Violet ever reads this, I hope things aren't the same. I hope she doesn't make Ajay call her every hour and a half. That's not healthy for either of them. I hope she can see herself more as the world sees her, how I saw her before I knew her. I know how hard it is. When you're apart, trust is hard sometimes. And even "gorgeous, perfect young women" need a solid reminder sometimes. The journey to loving oneself is the hardest and longest journey of all.

While some might judge Violet, her worry comes from her experience and knowledge of ship life. Ship moms like Violet—in romantic relationships with their babies' fathers—are the exception, not the rule. I feel grateful that I'm also in the exception category.

Single moms often deal with challenges such as financial strain, child care, fatigue, and loneliness, just to name a few.

A Scottish ship mom told me, "We did stay in contact for a while, but after he stopped answering my messages, I stopped sending them. If he doesn't want to know her, he doesn't deserve her."

"I wish I took more action and made his dad take more responsibility. I struggled as a single mom and financially. It made me sad to think my girl would not have a father," said a French ship mom.

In many of these cases, the paternal families have no idea that their ship-baby relatives exist. Some of these families go through their entire lives never knowing about their family member growing up elsewhere. One ship mom from the Philippines told me, "The father was already married with kids, so I didn't expect anything from him. I went through with the pregnancy anyway and gave birth alone. Afterwards, I sunk into a deep depression for four months. I did not talk. I only cried. I told myself I needed to be strong for my kids, and I forced myself to work." Some single moms don't have the luxury of taking a break, even when one is needed.

A Canadian ship mom said, "Being a single mom of twins is tough. Instead of having two parents with one baby, I am one parent with two babies. I have no regrets, though. Those kids are my whole world."

Being a single parent is challenging, but it can be a rewarding journey. I've seen these amazing moms embrace the lessons, develop a solid support system, and be empowered by their independence.

Many of the single ship moms also informed me that they were asked for paternity tests. One British ship mom told me, "I had to find the father on Facebook to tell him. He asked for a paternity test." An expectant father asking for a paternity test for the baby can be a tricky—and, in some cases, offensive—request for a pregnant woman. If a man wants to put his name on a birth certificate, shouldn't he be allowed to confirm that he is, in fact, the father? Many men think so and even feel it should be a mandatory practice.

So, what if the mother is not being honest about the father of her child? One German ship mom told me, "I'm living with my family, and they all believe that a Filipino is the father. But only my therapist knows about the true father."

If a mother deliberately gives false information that contributes to the establishment of paternity, she may be fined. It doesn't happen all that often, but in the small percentage of circumstances where it does, the results can be devastating. In paternity fraud, two men are actually defrauded: the biological father, who is not given a choice, and the alleged father, who is not given the truth. These men are often bewildered when they realize that the child they believed was theirs is not. The reasons why a woman would tell a man that he's the father when he isn't vary greatly depending on the circumstances. A woman could be seeking child support or could simply be wrong.

Apart from a paternity test, the other most common request from the ship dads was for an abortion. Like an unexpectedly pregnant mother, the father will experience many emotions when hearing the news. If the couple is in a relationship, a conversation is likely to be had, taking into consideration how he feels. But how much of a say should he get if there is no relationship?

"He was very angry when I told him," a Dominican ship mom told me. "He told me to abort it."

Obviously, men cannot compete with women when it comes to pregnancy because the woman carries the baby. In turn, if a woman goes ahead with the pregnancy that the father wants nothing to do with, should she still be able to come after him for financial support? Maybe legally, but the jury is still out on whether or not that's moral and right. One thing is for sure: there is a respectful and a disrespectful way to tell a partner you would like them to get an abortion.

"He denied the baby was his. He said I cheated. Told me to get an abortion." a Peruvian ship mom said. That is an example of what not to do.

I did interview a crew member who got pregnant on board and decided to abort the baby. We'll call her Patricia. An American, she was working as cruise staff on board when she got pregnant with a fellow crew member. Not ready to be a mother and only in her twenties, Patricia decided to have an abortion. She admits that she was in a privileged position to get off the ship and do that with no issues. She wanted to share her story because she didn't think the topic should be shied away from. Every woman decides what she wants to do with her own body, and if you take away the right to do it safely, women will find other ways.

In 2017, *The Royal Gazette* reported on a Filipina crew member who admitted to taking misoprostol on board to induce a miscarriage. She was given a three-month conditional discharge at the Supreme Court of Bermuda, the country in which the ship *Norwegian Dawn* was registered. Her partner, an Indian citizen who was also a crew member, was also given a three-month conditional discharge after he pleaded guilty to being an accessory, as he attempted to take the aborted fetus off the cruise liner in his rucksack.

In 2019, *The Sun* released a story with the clickbait headline "CRUISE HORROR Disney cruise ship entertainer gave herself illegal full-term abortion then hid STILL LIVING baby in a cupboard." The Brazilian crew member had bought abortion pills while the ship was in Mexico, then had a "secret illegal abortion in her cabin." Crew members ultimately found the woman bleeding to death. The baby later died, "hidden in a bag in a cupboard."

These are just two examples of countless stories of women who felt they had no choice but to take matters into their own hands and put their lives at risk.

While researching this book, I learned about Women on Waves (WOW), a Dutch non-governmental organization created to bring reproductive health services to countries where these are restricted. Unsafe or DIY abortions in regions where abortion is outlawed or restricted are a leading cause of maternal death. Once in international waters, WOW's medical personnel provide a range of reproductive health services that include medical abortion. The organization has faced considerable opposition, such as protesters chanting at its organizers, calling them Nazis, and even trying to tow the WOW vessel back out to sea, as shown in the 2014 documentary *Vessel*.[2]

Addressing the deeply rooted social, cultural, and economic barriers that make it more difficult for people to exercise their reproductive rights has been ongoing for years and continues to this day. Programs and services like WOW stand up for the principle that safe abortion is a human right. Every person who can become pregnant has the right to control their fertility and exercise reproductive autonomy. WOW continues to run today and has received more than one hundred thousand emails from women worldwide.

We were happy with our family trio. I didn't want to have another child, nor could we support another—physically or financially. Immediately, I knew I was going to get an abortion. Again, I called Ginnie and Chandra in tears—and not just because we had to cancel on the Hawksley Workman show we had tickets to that night. They provided me with all the proper information and who to contact. I cried about it once, but only once. If the timing and circumstances had been different, my choice might have been different.

The morning before I got my abortion, I was watching YouTube shorts and suddenly heard Donald Trump's grating voice saying, "The Democrats are the radical ones on this position because they support abortion up to and even beyond the ninth month . . . and even execution after birth."[3] I hung my head at the disinformation and made my way to the abortion clinic, scared that there might be protesters.

Mainly, I worried that I wouldn't be able to control my hormones and would start to argue with them.

Luckily, no protesters were there, and I was relieved. I later learned that protests were legally banned within forty metres of the clinic, which was nice to hear. The people at the clinic were warm, friendly, and caring. They also put in a new IUD for me. After my procedure, I didn't feel sad. I felt relieved. Even more so, I felt an overwhelming sense of pride and luck to be in Newfoundland and to be a Canadian. I felt so appreciative that I lived in a place where I could exercise my right to choose what I wanted to do with my own body. Further to that, I could do it in a medical environment with health-care workers, in a place that was safe and comfortable. If I had wanted to exercise that right while working on a cruise ship out of Florida, I would not have been able to do so. Rather, the choice would have been made for me by a regressive government.

Why would I share all this very personal information with you, opening myself up to judgment and criticism from not just the public but possibly also friends and family? Until now, only those two close friends and my sisters knew about my abortion.

This book about pregnancy features a bunch of women who found themselves pregnant and chose to have babies. I know that every woman on a cruise ship who gets pregnant has to weigh her options. Many, like Patricia, choose not to go forward with the pregnancy for any number of very valid reasons that, frankly, are nobody's business but theirs.

I wanted to add a personal perspective, for the women who chose to get an abortion while on board. I added it for all the women worldwide who wanted that choice but found that it was unavailable.

It seems to me that—for the majority of those who are anti-abortion—their caring stops after birth. I put myself out there like this to support women's inviolable autonomy over matters concerning their bodies and reproduction. Abortion is a medical procedure, and every woman should have the right to choose—for her body and her family.

I wanted to share my drinking problem for the same reason—to be real about something that impacts so many of us. Let's be honest, people. As a Newfoundlander and as a crew member, I was part of two groups that have a reputation for drinking hard. It's easy to hide in plain sight when you work in this industry or live in this place. Plus, it was hard not to write about this because it was during this writing process that I quit drinking. Although I'm nervous about communicating this so publicly, I think it gives me extra accountability and strengthens my commitment.

At first, an alcohol-free life seemed unnatural. But as time passes, it seems more obviously natural not to drink. The morbid truth is that it's only luck I am still alive and well after some of the messed-up situations I got myself in while drunk.

On one of my first social nights out after stopping, I drank a non-alcoholic beer. It went down nicely, so I quickly got another. I started chugging the second non-alcoholic beer like I had just hiked a mountain. Then I suddenly stopped, thinking, *What the hell am I doing?* Even the taste and smell of the non-alcoholic beer had struck something inside me and had me plowing them back, in search of a buzz I was not going to get. I wanted to get real with myself and acknowledge that I have a problem. I didn't bother with any non-alcoholic drinks after that.

It's not been easy to avoid drinking, but I feel a major sense of accomplishment and pride that I've gone this long. Sure, I still sometimes miss the buzz, but the next day, I'm always thankful to feel normal. I don't call myself "sober" because I am technically not. I thoroughly enjoy the Canadian legalization of marijuana, so one might call me "California sober."

Whatever you want to call it, I'm not drinking because it's what is best for me. I stay away from places where I would typically drink and plan activities that don't involve drinking. I am not saying I'll never have a drink again. Maybe I'll find a way to drink responsibly one day. But until then, I will be off the booze.

I do at least see myself—like my late grandmother Minnie Winsor—very late in my years, enjoying a couple of hot toddies and having a time. But, at least for now, I know I need to give up this one thing, for everything. This has been one of the hardest but best decisions I have ever made.

I once had the opinion that I was responsible for every single one of those blackout nights that left me traumatized because I had put myself in that position. I had to acknowledge my shame in order to accept and recover. My shame—a totally normal human emotion—was for myself. But then I would stop and think, *What about the person who thought it was okay to have sex with an unconscious person?*

The shame was also starting to build every time I let people get away with taking advantage of me. Although I am actively working on not drinking—thereby being able to ensure I'm not putting myself in these potentially harmful situations—some of those incidents never leave me. They are just flashes of memory in between blackness, but they're there, tormenting me.

These days, working in the literary industry, my events are much tamer. They start at seven in the morning and end at nine in the evening, unlike the music-industry events that started at nine in the evening and ended sometime the next day. When someone called about a big job opportunity in the music industry, I let them know I had no interest in applying and did confess that alcohol was a significant reason. I'm hitting almost a year alcohol-free and about to finally finish this project that has been a big part of my life for seven years.

These days, my definition of a great weekend doesn't include bars, binge drinking, or nursing a hangover. I am much more content with fuzzy blankets, a good book, and binge-watching reality TV. That said, there is no part of me that thinks I have alcohol, or my addictive personality, conquered. I don't want the added pressure of people thinking I'm some sort of role model for not drinking. I certainly don't have it all figured out and won't be leading a TED Talk on binge drinking and alcohol abuse anytime soon.

Although I wonder what level of backlash I'll receive for revealing so much about myself in such a public way, I still hope the good will outweigh the bad. In any case, writing the book has been therapeutic, and dreaming about it got me through some dark days. I feel more empowered, healed, and rooted in my life. I'm excited to close this chapter, and while I'm unsure what's next for me, I am not worried.

As long as I have Gabriel and Luiz with me, I know I can take on the world, which is the equivalent of writing a book if you ask me.

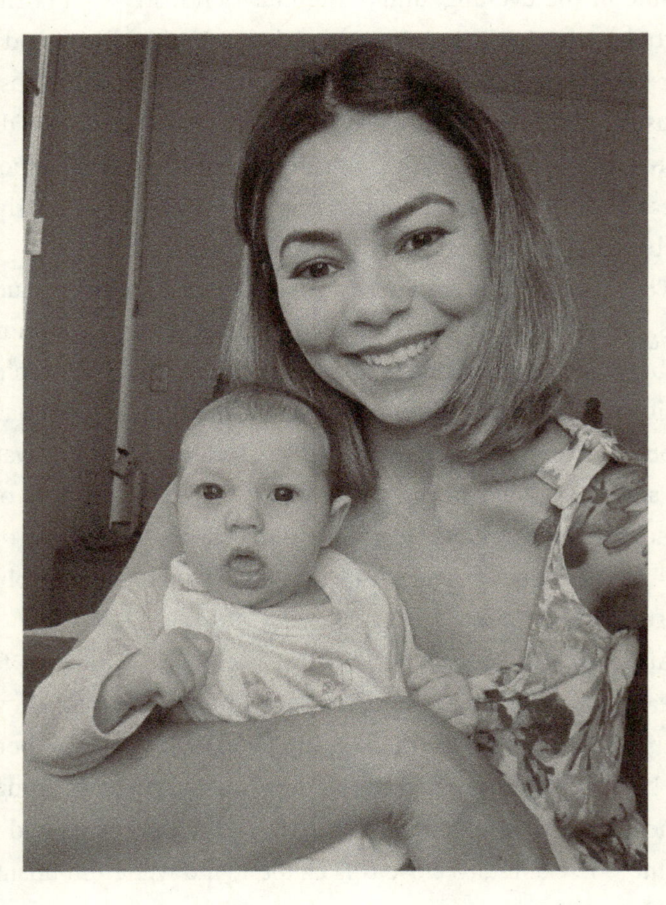

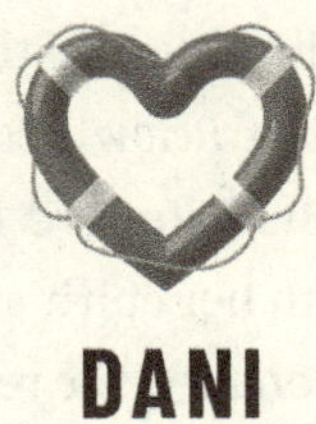

DANI

During the first years researching this book, my time was slim and my attention was scattered. But I still devoted time to read, watch, and listen to any and all things related to cruise ships and crew life. Because I struggled to find a hands-free minute for a physical book, I devoured audiobooks and other media. And I was beyond delighted to discover a television series, *Below Deck*, about crew living on board yachts. Bravo TV's popular American reality docuseries started in 2013 and chronicles the lives of crew who work and reside on board superyachts during charter season.

When I first joined a crew, I was sure that ship life would make for terrific reality TV. And I was right.

I was immediately hooked and convinced Luiz to watch it with me because there were many similarities to our cruise-ship experience. The show had grown into multiple spinoffs, including *Below Deck Mediterranean*, *Below Deck Sailing Yacht*, and *Below Deck Down Under*. We had a lot of catching up to do and binged the seasons easily. Thanks, pandemic! Every time a Canadian or Brazilian joined the cast, we would root for them amongst the crew and hope they represented our countries well.

After watching every iteration of the show, we had caught up to the current season of *Below Deck Sailing Yacht* and had been introduced to Brazilian steward Dani. It took only a few episodes to fall in love with her spirit and confidence. With her work-hard, play-hard personality, she reminded me of myself on ships. Like sweet Chef Kiko before her, she was a great rep for Brazilian *Below Deck* fans.

After the season was completed, I got news through my sister Sam, a fellow *Below Deck* follower, that there was a rumour Dani was pregnant. As soon as I heard this, my stomach flopped with excitement: I joked to Luiz that she would be in this book. He laughed but reminded me to shoot for the stars, to reach out anyway. Sure, she's a reality-show star, but you never know, right?

So how do you properly invite a reality star to be in your book when you have no money or contacts in reality TV? A cesspool at the worst of times and a saviour at the best of times, social media makes it possible for us little people to connect with famous folks. But like the letter I'd sent Daniel Johns in my early twenties, I expected that this letter would also go unanswered.

I started my Instagram DM with a Portuguese "Hi," hoping Dani would open it, read the beginning, and feel intrigued.

"Oi Dani! My name is Jen Winsor, and I am the author of the forthcoming book *Ship Moms*, which is a collection of true stories about crew who got pregnant while working on board. Writing you today wondering if you may be available and interested in doing a virtual interview with me. Like you, I got pregnant while working on board with a younger man that I had just met. I was 35, he was 23 and Brazilian!"

It was December, so I ended the message with *Feliz Natal!*—"Merry Christmas" in Portuguese—crossed my fingers, and pressed send. One night a week or so later, probably watching *Below Deck* with Luiz, my phone pinged, and there was Dani's response: *I would love to!*

I was so thrilled I was teary-eyed. When I held up the message for Luiz to see, he smiled and shrugged.

"See?" he said, as if he had known she'd agree all along.

I am honoured that Dani was willing to share her story with me. Our first interview session was in February 2022, via Zoom. She has almost one hundred and sixty thousand Instagram followers, and you can find articles about her in *People* and *Us Weekly*. I even found a *Daily Mail* article that was simply about her getting a new pixie haircut! Dani is a public figure with fans and, sadly, some online enemies who make moving through life a little more challenging at times. This life in the public eye is a far stretch from growing up in the melting pot of one of the world's most populous cities with her two brothers and her single mom.

Dani's mom is the second youngest of eleven Indigenous siblings who grew up in the northeast countryside of Brazil's São Paulo state. They worked on the family farm, picking and planting beans instead of studying at school. Dani's grandmother was a spiritual woman who, following the culture of her tribe, spoke with the land, the animals, and even the spirits of her ancestors. Dani's mother and her family shared the responsibilities of the home and farmland. However, being adventurous like her future daughter, Dani's mom—beautiful and then just nineteen—couldn't wait to move to the booming, cosmopolitan city of São Paulo, with all of its possibilities and opportunities. Her kind-natured spirit and her rural roots made her gullible and easily taken advantage of. She got pregnant with Dani soon after arriving. Years later, two brothers were added to the family.

Dani had a humble upbringing and spent most of her time helping raise her brothers and get them to and from school. She calls her childhood "boring," yet she grew up in one of the most dangerous neighbourhoods in one of the most dangerous cities. It was—and still is—the sort of place where you don't take your phone out of your pocket or wear fancy jewelry or shoes because you would be robbed by looters lurking on every corner.

"I grew up in one of the worst neighbourhoods in São Paulo and went to the worst school," Dani said, admitting she had been desensitized to guns and violence. "I remember seeing guys with guns all the time. My mom would always say, 'Just be friendly. But don't ignore them. Don't be rude.'" That was until Dani hit puberty and the gunmen started looking at her new curves with different eyes. Her mom moved her and her brothers out of that neighbourhood soon after.

Of course, growing up in São Paulo wasn't all bad. Dani grew up with street smarts and intuition, which she would have never gained while living in suburbia. She was a hustler doing whatever she could, selling trinkets, erasers, and pencils.

At eighteen she started working at McDonald's. One day she found herself immediately smitten by a new employee, Felipe. After watching him get his uniform squared away, without even speaking to him, Dani told her co-worker, "That guy's going to be my boyfriend." She could feel his smile, warmth, and charisma across the room. Once they talked, they hit it off immediately, and as Dani had predicted, he became her boyfriend.

A couple of years passed, and while Dani and Felipe's teenage relationship was going well, they started to have adult conversations about what they wanted out of life. Dani had always had a fire inside her to see the world and experience everything life had to offer before settling down to be a mother. Pursuing travel and tourism, she got a scholarship to one of the best hospitality universities in São Paulo and started studying. Felipe had dreamt of working in the police force and making a family in Brazil. As he worked toward joining the Military Police of São Paulo State, Dani scored a job on a cruise ship and her first ever plane ticket out of Brazil. The couple decided to break up.

Dani is unsure how she passed the English test to get that first job on the *Monarch of the Seas* Royal Caribbean cruise ship. She recalls her first day and how she didn't know the English word for "tray"—not good for an on-board waitress! Not only were the guests all American with their particular slang, but the crew was made up of dozens of nationalities who spoke English with their accents. Like most new-hire cruise crew, Dani found the first few weeks on board gruelling and was unsure of what she had gotten herself into. But after some time, her English improved, and she started enjoying the crew life, learning a lot about the world and herself, which was precisely what she had been looking for. Her time on board the cruise ship was short lived, as she signed off after a few months, but it was official: the travel bug had bitten Dani and would change her entire life.

While home in Brazil, Dani accompanied a friend to a screening process for Emirates Airlines. Dani knew nothing about Dubai or being a flight attendant but figured, why not tag along for the experience? After it was confirmed that Dani had ticked the two most important boxes—that she was a fluent English speaker and tall enough to reach the overhead compartment handles—she was asked to return the next day. She went home, Googled "Dubai," and took out her most professional-looking outfit in preparation. To Dani's surprise, she passed the complex screening process and started as a flight attendant for the airline. This was the beginning of three years of travelling the world in the skies. Her new position was fun and glamorous—and on her days off, she would visit countries she hadn't been to yet. While she still worked hard, the job wasn't as demanding or as crazy as the cruise-ship work had been.

While working in Dubai, Dani hit it off with a handsome Irish chef. Like her, he was focused on seeing the world and suggested they try yachting for a summer in France. Who would not want to spend the summer in France, yachting with a handsome Irishman? So, with no experience, Dani flew to France and started "dock walking," an industry term yachties use to describe walking the docks and networking for jobs. "Yachtie" is a name for people who work on yachts. It sometimes has a negative connotation—think "carney"—so don't use that term around crew loosely.

Dani had no experience on yachts, but her cruise- and flight-crew resumé gave her a leg up, and she got job offers on two boats immediately. She chose a fifty-five-metre doing housekeeping because it paid slightly more. As they had anticipated, the Irish chef didn't get hired on the same boat, and they eventually went their separate ways.

Slowly but surely working her way out of the laundry, Dani grew to love the job and luxury and continued on yachts non-stop. Like many crew members, she would say, "One more contract, and I am done" but keep returning after every vacation. After five years and a hard breakup with an on-board first officer, she made her way to Madrid. The plan was to receive a beauty-therapy diploma after a year and then move to Australia, her dream destination, to settle down. Right before the plan was executed, she flew home to Brazil to see her family and let them know.

During this vacation back home, Dani agreed to meet up with her former teenaged McDonald's love, Felipe. Like their first meeting years before, he drew Dani in again like a magnet. She swooned over how he wasted no time telling her how he had always longed for her, recalling little details about her that he loved, like the one piece of straight hair in her naturally curly hair. He was the calm sea to her spinning whirlpool, and while he was still the caring, silly person she had met years ago, now he was a grown man passionate about his dream job in the police force and knew what he wanted in life.

Dani fell head over heels, and her Madrid-Australia plan quickly went out the window while she secured a beauty-therapy job there in São Paulo. They immediately fell deeply in love. Both now in their thirties, they were ready to finally settle down and start making a life together in Brazil. Within months, they had moved in together and were engaged. Because they shared the significance of having birthdays on January and February 17, they decided on May 17 of the following year for the wedding.

Exactly one year and one month before the nuptials, in pursuit of a suspect who ran from a stop in a tight alley in a *favela* in the south of São Paulo, Felipe was shot on duty. A sad and eerie coincidence, it was April 17.

Both Dani and Felipe's mom discovered the shooting when Felipe's Facebook profile picture was posted on the local news, which stated that a police officer had been shot. With all his social-media photos plastered on the screen, the news satellite image focused on the crime scene, following the police cars flooding the alleys. Felipe was taken to the Albert Einstein hospital but tragically succumbed to his injuries. He was only thirty-two years old. For Dani, her life—and the number seventeen, their number—would never be the same.

Due to the pandemic, the usual process to honour a police officer could not be performed. There would be no gun salute or wake with the participation of representatives from all police headquarters in the city. Instead, when Felipe was laid to rest in the São Paulo Military Police Mausoleum, police squad cars lined the street with their sirens turned on. Paying respect to their colleague, the police saluted and stood at attention. All 645 cities in the state of São Paulo did the same. Felipe's mother received the Brazilian flag, folded in a box. He had been a proud member of the police force for four years.

Feeling shocked and defeated, Dani was left in severe grief. She and Felipe had only just started their life together. She had felt safe with him and sure of their life plan. After his death, she couldn't speak of Felipe or look at photos of him as it would lead to uncontrollable crying fits and physical pain. Worrying her friends and family, she stopped eating and got frighteningly thin. She then turned to alcohol for comfort, which inevitably led to more destructive behaviour, going as far as getting into fights in bars. She was deep into self-destruct mode and didn't care what happened to her.

Three months later, lost and seeking any escape from her despair, Dani sought a way out of where she was. Randomly, she signed up for the opportunity to be cast on Bravo TV's *Below Deck*. Like I'd felt when I sent her my DM, she didn't think anything would come of it. When she watched the show and saw the *Below Deck* casting call on social media, she filled out a form and uploaded a photo. When contacted for an interview, Dani was at a very low point and thought, *Well, a reality show is completely out of left field. I could do this and remove myself from here. I can be a different person, living a different life.* This reality show was a new world where she could act normal and not be absorbed by grief.

After countless Zoom interviews with producers and executives and a thorough background check, Dani was asked to join the show as a stewardess in its *Sailing Yacht* series. Unlike many other reality stars, she didn't prepare for her term on the show with coaching on how to get more airtime, how to behave in front of the camera, or how to conduct herself in the public eye. Dani thought she would take on this new adventure as she had taken on every opportunity that had ever presented itself: by winging it and hustling.

Because the season was filmed during the pandemic, there was a lot of pre-preparation and isolation before Dani and her cast mates joined the boat. As soon as she stepped on board *Parsifal III*, the cameras were on her. She was miked and stayed that way twenty-four hours a day.

Having an entirely separate crew of camera and sound technicians day and night was an adjustment for all the cast members. The cast initially felt awkward and wanted to say hello or apologize if they bumped into production staff, but the film crew didn't engage. They were lovely people—always very professional and polite—but they had a role to play in the show, and the cast were to talk to producers only.

As time passed, the cast members learned why. The film crew slowly became like furniture around the room: the cast knew they were there but didn't think about them anymore. The crew were constantly present, filming every minute—even of crew doing laundry for five hours or eating cereal—hoping to catch any random moment of reality TV gold. Sometimes, forgetting where she was, Dani would catch herself daydreaming or picking at her teeth in front of a camera, and would giggle at being caught.

Dani immediately hit it off with her fellow cast and crew mates, and fans weren't at all disappointed in the change in the ship's crew, which arguably made for a much more compelling season than the previous one.

For any readers not familiar with the show or this season, let me give you some notable points of reference. The ship's crew signs on, and First Officer promptly hooks up with Deckhand; the crew parties in the hot tub; they do an eighties night for the guests; Chief Stewardess and Chef are at odds over serving the guests meals; six-foot-nine Deckhand is too tall to fit in his bunk; the crew parties and plays Truth or Dare; they do a drag show for the guests; Deckhand and Stewardess fight over First Officer; Dani starts hooking up with the tall Deckhand; the crew parties;

they do a casino night for the guests; the anchor tangles and high winds keep deck crew busy; First Officer hooks up with another Stewardess; they do a murder-mystery night for the guests; there is an STD scare; yachtie peers come on board for a charter. And if all that was not enough, the yacht crashes into the dock—a *Below Deck* first.

The tall deckhand was immediately attracted to Dani's accent, but soon he also noticed her friendly nature and how she was a hard worker and never involved in drama. Dani, on the other hand, didn't think of him romantically at first. One night, while playing Truth or Dare, he was asked who he would choose from the crew if he had his pick. He said Dani. After they share their first kiss during a dare in the game, Dani starts to feel him as well. After that night, the pair were consistently hooking up. Initially casual, their relationship became more serious over the filming, making them the "couple of the season."

Although Dani liked him and was having fun, she wasn't sure they were looking for the same thing. At just twenty-four, the guy had never been in a relationship longer than three weeks—a red flag for her. With their nine-year age difference, he also seemed a little too young for her, and, honestly, the last thing on her mind was starting a long-term relationship. That said, Dani was open about being ready to settle down and have a family. The show, whether strategically or not, played her saying so multiple times.

"You make me feel like I'm the most amazing person in the world," she told him in one episode. "But I just don't see how this could actually work. That's what you get when you get with thirty-plus-year-old women who have no time to waste."

For anyone who watched the season, you know Dani also had moments in which she wanted to call it quits. She later admitted in podcasts that she was regularly having panic attacks behind the scene. In one confessional, she said, "How did I get here? I'm in my thirties. I do like my job, but it's not my career. I'm hooking up with a twenty-year-old boy, I'm having fights with a crew member, and I'm still grieving over the love of my life."

As if things couldn't get more complex, the deckhand then tells her that he thinks he may have an STD.

"I'm thinking I'm having fun and enjoying myself, and then there you go, with this serious shit," Dani yelled after he told her about his issue.

It was then that Dani told her chief stew that she wanted to leave *Parsifal III* and go home.

In this real moment, Dani felt she was being punished. She felt she should return to the depressed Dani she had been months before—sad and mourning. She was enjoying herself too much in this bubble where she could act like everything was okay, and it was making her feel very guilty. Thanks to a helpful chat and a good night's sleep, Dani knew she needed to continue and finish what she had started. Luckily, as the viewers learned, the deckhand's symptoms turned out not to be an STD but just chafing.

After the season ended, the ship's crew signed off, and interviews were all done. Due to the pandemic, everyone needed to quarantine in a hotel in Croatia for two weeks before travelling. After filming wrapped, Dani and the deckhand spent a couple of days together before going into their individual isolation rooms to prepare for travel to their next destinations.

In isolation, Dani started researching and preparing for her next chapter: nursing school and a move to her dream country, Australia. She noticed that her breasts were feeling heavy, and she felt strange. When her period was a couple of days late, she ordered a pregnancy test online. It was delivered the next day, and, to her surprise, the test strip confirmed she was expecting. She didn't believe it so ordered three more, this time making sure to buy different brands just in case. All three came back positive. Dani was pregnant.

While this wasn't the ideal situation, she was ready to be a mother, and—if this was how the universe would make her one—she wanted to make it work. She contacted the deckhand immediately and told him straight: "I am pregnant, and you are the father."

He reacted as most twentysomethings who have only been in a three-week relationship would react. He was shocked but somewhat supportive during that first conversation. That was until they spoke again, and this time his tone was different. He had changed his mind.

"I want a paternity test," he told her.

Dani told him he was the only person she had been with, and she found his request a little hard to process.

Why does a woman get angry when a man asks for this confirmation? Because asking a woman for this says that the father doesn't trust her and thinks the baby isn't his. It makes the assumption that the woman is a liar and has stepped out on the man. Maybe it's a projection. Many cheaters are paranoid that their partners are cheating on them. If a man's primary thought when his partner gets pregnant is "gotta make sure it's mine," there are likely going to be problems in that relationship. In fact, there already are.

At the same time, asking a woman to take a paternity test to ensure you don't raise a child that isn't yours is not bad. It's a responsible thing to do when done respectfully. But it's a very complicated question to ask a pregnant woman who knows damn well whether or not she has had sex with someone else. Only a terrible person would lie to a man about the paternity of their child, right? Did the deckhand suddenly think Dani was a terrible person?

She reacted to this as most hormonal woman would—emotionally. She angrily told him, "No problem," but if he wanted a test, he had to pay for it. She let him know he was welcome to stay in touch.

This was the start of a rocky road to come. After many tears, Dani concluded that everything happens for a reason and that this pregnancy would move forward with or without the deckhand's involvement. She didn't know where or how, but she knew she could do it.

With her travel career no longer an option, Dani had to decide where she would make a home for herself and her child, and she had to figure out how to make money in these trying times. The pandemic had hit her homeland hard. Behind only the United States and Russia, Brazil had the third-highest number of confirmed COVID cases and the sixth-highest death toll globally. Although Brazil was her birthplace, she knew it wasn't safe, and the leadership, or lack thereof, of conservative and controversial president Jair Bolsonaro—who spent the pandemic perpetuating conspiracy theories and downplaying the seriousness of COVID[5]—

wasn't helping. This guy made Donald Trump look good. I wish that were a joke, but it isn't. Dani decided going home to Brazil was not an option.

After much thought, she followed her gut and decided to pursue the dream of settling in Australia and studying nursing. Australia was a safe, stable country with a friendly, relaxed culture, beautiful landscapes, and bustling cities. If she continued to pursue this path, it would provide a better future for herself and her "soon-to-be" daughter, who would automatically be an Australian citizen due to Dani's permanent-resident status at the time of birth.

Two days after leaving quarantine, Dani secured a job as a beauty therapist in Sydney while also enrolling in nursing school. She worked and studied hard, and normally had twelve-hour days. She knew nobody there but, luckily, found a solid support system, mainly in her team of female colleagues. Nobody knew about Dani's pregnancy apart from her spa co-workers, close friends, and family, on whom she leaned for support during this difficult time. Luckily, her manager turned into such a close friend that she ended up being with Dani in the delivery room. If she had gotten a different job and had not met these supportive women, she's unsure how she would have made it through the pregnancy.

While Dani was at work one day, six months pregnant, someone who recognized her from *Below Deck* took a photo—without her knowledge—of her and her growing belly. The whistle-blowing photographer then shared the photo with gossip pages online. Dani didn't get to share the news with the world as she had wanted to because somebody else did, and the story blew up.

Soon enough, Instagram started spinning with the newest reality-show drama, making *Below Deck* fans speculate about who the father was. The keyboard crusaders all gave their opinions and stirred the pot vigorously, posting questions and theories on Dani, the deckhand, and cast members' online photos. The Insta-drama hit the roof when a fan commented on the deckhand's profile that he was "gross" for not taking responsibility for his child. This was followed by the deckhand's mother commenting, "Gross is a woman who uses a man because she's so desperate to be a mom."[6] As the pot was about to boil over, the fans and gossip lovers ate up all the drama.

On June 22, 2021, the *Below Deck Sailing Yacht* cast came together virtually on *Watch What Happens Live with Andy Cohen*, to break down everything that had happened during the show's second season. The deckhand, whom everyone wanted to grill, was noticeably absent. The reunion cast awkwardly answered Andy's questions, which put them on the spot about embarrassing things they had done on the show.

Dani received congratulations on her pregnancy, but the vibe quickly shifted when Andy asked if she was in touch with the deckhand or his family. She told Andy about the social-media backlash with his mom and the nasty messages she had received, which insinuated that she had tricked the deckhand into impregnating her.

"I say during the whole season that I want to be a mom and have a family.... That was my plan. That was my vision. I would not choose to move to a new country where I don't know anybody and choose to have a child with a 24-year-old boy that I barely knew . . . I did not plan that. I am just going with this now and

I am sure my little baby girl is going to be amazing." Dani's voice cracked as she talked to Andy. "He hasn't supported me at all in any way. He thinks it is not his child and he doesn't want to have anything to do with it."[7]

Andy said he was sorry to hear the news, and the cast gave their opinions on the situation. Regarding the deckhand's unwillingness to accept that the baby was his, one cast member expressed revulsion and exasperation. Another, whose father had chosen not to be in his life, said that he had lost all respect for his former cast mate.

Dani reminded her crew mates and viewers that the deckhand wasn't there to speak for himself, which I thought was kind and generous. She told me later she had done this for her daughter. She said she wanted her future child to only hear the facts about the situation and not as much opinion. Every story has two sides, after all. Dani's mother never spoke ill of her father, who abandoned them, and she planned to do the same. Even when Dani grew up and saw her father for who he was, her mom still never spoke poorly of him. She just reminded her daughter that he was the only father she had. Like Dani, her daughter will eventually make up her own mind about how she feels about her father and the story of how she came to be.

After the deckhand declined to do the reunion with the cast, to the fans' delight, producers arranged a separate interview with Andy Cohen, where he addressed the speculation that he was the baby's father.

"If that is my child, I want *everything* and *anything* to do with that child's life,"[8] the deckhand said in the interview. He stayed planted in his denial, asking for a DNA test before he would ever acknowledge his paternity.

Dani tried her best not to get too wrapped up in the online drama, instead focusing on taking care of her body and her growing belly. She worked up until two days before giving birth, and then Miss Lilly came into the world quickly, with Dani pushing for only twenty minutes.

She posted on her Instagram account, captioning a photo of the newborn's little hand. "She is here. She is perfect. And we are trying to figure this thing out. We both healthy and happy. Thank you for all the support. Will post more once mummy had some rest."[9]

Because Dani had practically raised her younger brothers from birth, she had felt very prepared to be a mother. But nothing could have readied her for the reality of the coming days. She pushed through those first weeks as best she could. Her body was recovering from the birth, she struggled with breastfeeding, and she had nursing-school exams set for a week after the delivery. During a practical exam, she was so laser-focused on taking vital signs properly that she didn't notice the two wet circles forming over her leaking breasts. Sleep deprived, she just shrugged and laughed it off, not caring what anyone thought. As all women who have experienced these post–baby delivery weeks know, Dani was hanging on by a thread, trying to keep her baby and herself healthy.

On June 18, 2021, four weeks after the baby's birth, the deckhand posted this on his Instagram: "There's a lot of gossip about my social media silence so I think it's time to clear the air. While others are off chasing their 15 minutes of fame, I am working on a yacht in Central America . . . [I'm] heartbroken to have to hear about the baby's birth on social media and read headlines, like, 'Dani Soares Says Her Baby's Father Doesn't Want Anything to Do With It.' All I can say is if it's mine, I want to be involved 100 [per cent] . . . As someone who grew up with parents who weren't together, I wouldn't wish that on any child. Not looking for a pity party. Just want everyone to know how strongly I feel about this, especially the haters who are so sure I am neglecting my responsibility. No one wants to know more than me if this is my baby girl!" [10]

While the caveman theory of newborns looking like their dads so that fathers recognize their offspring isn't scientifically proven, anyone with functioning eyes and half a brain can see that Lilly was the deckhand's daughter.

Dani says social media, Instagram in particular, quickly became both a negative and positive. People sent her encouraging messages, sharing their stories about their amazing single moms and how things would get better. These gave her strength, which was very appreciated on those particularly hard days. On the other hand, she also received messages telling her she was awful for bringing a baby into the world without its father, for taking advantage of a man by tricking him into getting her pregnant, and for playing a victim because she "asked for it."

Dani responded to a few of the trolls but learned quickly that there is no debating with these "fans." Trolls don't want to know the facts or your side of the story. Using inflammatory messages, they just want to get a rise out of you, to provoke you into responding. Their reasons could include revenge, attention seeking, boredom, or—in the case of the truly messed up—personal amusement.

While some *Below Deck* fans still supported the deckhand online, I can only imagine how much harassment from reality-show lovers he must have received. Fans and several of his cast members called for him to deal with the possibility that the child was his.

The deckhand responded that he was actively looking to take a paternity test, stating: "I know paternity test kits are available at drugstores but the goal is for us to take the tests together instead of shipping saliva samples around the world." [11]

In my first interview with Dani, we talked about the deckhand, and I asked her how she thought things would play out with the paternity. She told me she assumed that when it was confirmed he was indeed the father, he would write a fluffy social-media post backtracking and deflecting from his previous stance. On January 19, 2022, not three weeks later, the deckhand captioned an Instagram photo of himself back on, looking out at the water. The highlights of what he wrote in that post what would appear in *Us Weekly* on February 22, 2022:

> "*A new year in 2022 begins with high ambitions and positivity . . . My silence on social media has been intentional and much needed. I used that time to focus on what was important to me and my mental health . . . I'm happy and proud to say sweet and beautiful Lilly Rose is my daughter . . . Dani and I have been working and communicating together to the best of our ability; given Dani is a full time mother and worker, and I being gone for extended periods of time not knowing when*

I will step back on land. This is imperative for the sake of our daughter as she needs both parents in her life." [12]

Dani couldn't help but get annoyed and then laugh at a reference to them co-parenting in his initial post because there was no sharing of the duties of raising Lilly. He did edit out that part after the fact, but thanks to social-media screenshots, the initial message will live on. Dani has gotten messages from women saying mean things and implying that she is keeping Lilly from her father. She doesn't bother responding and tries to keep positive for her daughter. She can't help but wonder: if this pregnancy and baby weren't so public, would he have completely disappeared like so many other ship and yacht dads?

The truth is that since testing confirmed Lilly is the deckhand's daughter, he has started talking to her on the phone occasionally. Dani welcomes calls on Monday and Wednesdays, but he is busy, so it's just a few times per month. The deckhand said he had started a college fund and asked for Dani's address to send something, but a gift has yet to arrive at the time of this writing. Dani admits she's still not much of a fan of talking to him but, for Lilly, will always pick up the phone if he calls.

Dani takes full responsibility for everything she said on the show and how she acted. While she may be a little embarrassed by some of it, she says that what you see is how it was. While reality shows are sometimes accused of not portraying things accurately, Dani told me she feels she was accurately portrayed. Apart from that one line she said once or twice but the media kept playing over and over: she was over thirty and wanted to have babies.

While that was true, she was referring to the life she had left behind. She dreamt of her late fiancé, Felipe; of a beautiful wedding on the beach; and of having babies and showing them the world. But that was a dream and not the reality she was living, even if it was an escape from reality.

Having a child was not Dani's new mission, but a reality-show's job is to entertain the viewer, so the show's producers included Dani's every comment about babies during the season, conveniently setting up tension for the pregnancy that would be revealed during the reunion. She hadn't planned to be a single mom with a twentysomething guy she hardly knew, but it didn't matter. Life happens and Dani was on board for the ride, clinging on with both hands.

Dani herself knows who her father is but doesn't really "know" her father. He never really treated her like a daughter or prioritized her in any way. Although she has him as a friend on Facebook, he doesn't even wish her happy birthday when Facebook reminds him. Although he's now a grandfather, that hasn't changed.

Dani also didn't have a relationship with her paternal grandmother, a woman who—like Lilly's paternal grandmother—loudly denied that her son had anything to do with their mother. Sadly, she passed before Dani ever got to meet her. That said, Dani has no hatred toward her father and even goes as far as to say, "If he ever loses all of his favourite kids and needs me, I will be there for him."

During my second interview with Dani in March 2022, she told me that the deckhand has never apologized for denying Lilly initially. She also said that his mother hasn't apologized for implying that her son was tricked into getting someone pregnant or for calling her granddaughter's mom "gross" on social media. Dani says her door is open if they want to form more of a relationship with Lilly, but she won't force it. Dani doesn't want her daughter to grow up and feel like she isn't wanted. She hopes to find a way to help Lilly understand that the opinions of her father and his family have nothing to do with her. The goal is to make Lilly know that she's loved—and that she was and will always be wanted. If her father and his family aren't engaged, then it's nothing to do with Lilly. It's all to do with them.

Overall, Dani feels fortunate for how things turned out. They certainly could have gone better in some respects but worse in others. When we first chatted, she planned to stay in Australia, finish school, and work as a nurse. She looked forward to raising Lilly in a safe country and a culture of outdoorsy people blessed with a sunny, warm, dry climate. Dani feels that she might not even be here right now if it weren't for Lilly. Her destructive path of not taking care of herself was now not an option. Lilly gave Dani a reason to live. She gave Dani the happiness and purpose she thought she had lost.

Dani says she still thinks about Felipe every day. Some days, every hour. When something very good or bad happens, she thinks of him and tells him that aloud. When planning how they would conquer life together, they talked intensely about how much they loved each other and how happy they were. Dani acknowledges that there had been no unanswered questions or things left on the table when he passed. Nothing was unsaid or unplanned. There were just the things they didn't get to do. She doesn't feel they could have done anything differently because they achieved everything they had planned, even if Felipe's life was cut too short doing what he loved.

Dani can't help but sometimes think about how she got pregnant very soon after he passed and harbours guilt over the joy her new daughter brings her. Does Felipe watch over her and Lilly begrudgingly? Deep down, Dani knows Felipe has given his love and blessing. He knew more than anyone how much Dani wanted to settle down and be a mother. He knew every single thing Dani wanted in life. He knew all her secrets, and she, his.

Chatting with Dani again in the fall of 2024, she let me know that after much work, as a single mom, she had graduated with a bachelor of nursing degree. That is no small feat. She had been working as a nurse for six months, and with money finally coming in, she can pay the bills. They can now afford to eat out once a week, and she can buy little things that Lilly wants. It's a common misconception that all reality stars are wealthy people drowning in brand deals and giveaways. Dani is not rich and works very hard every day to provide for her girl. She's applying for her Australian citizenship this year but admits that she is lonely a lot and considering moving back to Brazil to be close to her mother and family.

When asked if she still watches *Below Deck*, she laughed and said, "I don't watch the show anymore."

Dani told me that sweet Lilly, now three years old, has started calling every man she comes across "Dad." Even random men on the street. Months back Dani contacted the deckhand and told him she'd like him to call at least once a week so his daughter would know who he was and so that they could form a bond, even if distantly. He called for a few weekends, which was appreciated, but then they had a frustrating call that had to be cut short because Lilly was sick. He was clearly annoyed by this. Even when Dani messaged to tell him sorry, Lilly was simply too sick to sit and chat. He saw the message but never responded, and Dani hasn't heard from him since.

Dani tried her best to keep him in Lilly's life, but it can't be forced. "It's not my job anymore," she said. "He can facilitate if he wants it."

She didn't ask for money; she just asked him to keep in touch. I'm sure she doesn't want to experience any more disappointment for herself or her daughter. No one in the deckhand's family, including his mother, Lilly's grandmother, have reached out to be in Lilly's life. Dani never did get an apology from his mother for her social-media comments. She likely never will.

Dani still thinks about Felipe a lot. "I feel robbed of a future I could have had," she told me. "I would have had my life partner, whom I will never find again." Dani doesn't think much about finding a new partner. She went out on a few dates with a guy who seemed promising, but it went nowhere fast after he cancelled on a date because he was "too hungover."

Dani feels like she'll never find love again. When I asked her why, she simply said, "Because nobody is Felipe." She says she was lucky to find her special person and have him for the amount of time she did. She thinks she lost the one big love of her life. She still keeps his photo up and can now look at it and enjoy it without getting upset.

Dani has also started gravitating to the number seventeen again. She thanks therapy for these healthy steps forward. When she is looking for an answer, it often seems that the number seventeen will pop up, confirming that it's the right choice.

Here's hoping that Dani meets the most amazing person. And maybe he'll be wearing a shirt with a vibrant number seventeen on it! That way, she'll know Felipe is watching over her and Lilly and sending his blessings. He sounds like a guy who would want the love of his life to love and be loved again in hers.

I struggled with writing this book at times, and almost stopped. When I kept working and couldn't see the finish line, I started to panic. But I was able to fight the panic because of the women, the ship moms. They gave me purpose. They shifted my focus when I needed it most, and the perspective I got from them was immeasurable.

At the beginning of the process, I was dating a much younger man whom I believed was way out of my league. I was self-conscious about myself. I lost an unhealthy amount of weight quickly and spent countless hours comparing myself to women online who were twenty years younger than me. The photos I posted were heavily filtered and Facetuned, and I wouldn't be caught dead not wearing makeup. I wanted to look younger, thinner, better than I thought I was. I was taking myself and life way too seriously.

In the following years, with inspiration from this project—the women and their stories—I started to feel more self-assured again.

My mojo started to creep back in.

When my confidence came back, to my surprise, I had gained even more spunk. I had finally grown a backbone as well.

Upon finishing my book, I posted a quick teaser message on my social media with a makeup-free, unfiltered selfie. Not thinking twice about my appearance is significant progress for me.

Coming to terms with my mental health and working through Gabriel's diagnosis has also been a journey. For a while, I was experiencing intense mood swings and low self-esteem. I was getting stressed out or angry easily—and maybe worst of all, dissociation. I was almost in a defeated daze, living in my head outside my immediate surroundings. I needed to work on my own mental health in order to better keep it together for Gabriel. Thanks to therapy and medication, I feel much better. Thank you, Lexapro!

Knowing what I know now, it's no surprise that my boy has hyperactive and impulsive ADHD. This condition is often seen in families with addiction problems. I try my best every day to break cycles and work on myself for him. I am now trying to look at the positives as well. As was pointed out once by my awesome "cousin-sister" Jodie, Gabriel and I can use our abundant energy, spontaneity, conversational skills, and hyperfocus to our advantage.

When Gabriel was four, he was obsessed with AC/DC, Jack Black, and rock music. He would take his guitar everywhere and play for people, telling them he wanted to "melt their faces." He only knew five chords but was so charming that he amazed people. Video evidence of him jamming "TNT" with bluegrass group High & Lonesome in Bannerman Park is available online for your enjoyment 'cause it's way too cute. (Apologies for my shrill voice when laughing/crying in the video.)

These days Gabriel loves Minecraft and wants to shave his head bald—not fully bald but a cul-de-sac, to look like his beloved grandfather Poppy Winsor and Unspeakable, a YouTuber Gabriel likes. He's not in many activities because, frankly, we haven't been able to afford it, so friends are a little scarce. But we're working on that.

I have no idea what's in store for Gabriel's future, but I'm not as scared as I once was. He is a bright and silly boy who recently freaked me out with his math skills, doing things I could never have done at his age. I see the progress and the "superpowers" in him—and in myself.

Today, there are more good days than "not good" days. It's easy to dwell on negativity when things are hard. After these past seven years of parenting while also working on this book, I'm not afraid to say how proud of myself I am. If this book entertains—and lessens the loneliness of—even one person, then mission accomplished! I sought to do that for myself, and I can only dream that this book will do the same for someone else.

Our sweet ship-baby boy, although living in Canada, is proud to be half-Brazilian, and he celebrates that part of himself. He loudly and proudly sings the Portuguese version of "Happy Birthday"—"Parabéns pra Você"—at every birthday party and wears a Brazilian soccer jersey most days. While he hasn't travelled to Brazil since he was just under two years old, we plan to visit soon. I know the trip will be a whole new and exciting experience now that Gabriel is older.

Our last visit there, to see the most welcoming family, was incredible, and we cannot wait to return. I fell in love with Guaraná pop, Havaianas flip-flops, cracking thunder, and drinking in public—but not too many Caipirinhas or Cachaça shots! I loved *churrasco*, Brazilian barbecue, so don't let that scene from the *Bridesmaids* movie scare you. The coarse rock-salt cooking method is amazing and doesn't give you the poops. Admittedly, I was a little nervous about Brazilian bathrooms, because you can't throw paper in the toilet, but I loved the bidets so much that we now have one in our bathroom at home.

There is so much to love about Brazil. The diversity, music, food, culture, and stunning scenery are just a few. I love the people: most seem to be good-looking, funny, and friendly, with a knack for putting things in a particular way that is either very mindful or hilarious. While many of the funny expressions are racy, the best ones are beautiful, like "flower of the skin," or *saudade*, which is like a feeling of "longing." My personal favourite would be *dar à luz*. Directly translated, this means "giving to light." An example would be, "Oh, you should see the babies! She gave light to twins!"

I think "giving light" for "giving birth" is such a great way to say what a woman has done for the world by giving life to a human being. It is, in fact, magical. It's a miracle. Every time a baby is presented to the world, it guarantees that life goes on. Although Gabriel is a firecracker, he is the sweet light of my life, and I am most honoured to be his ship mom.

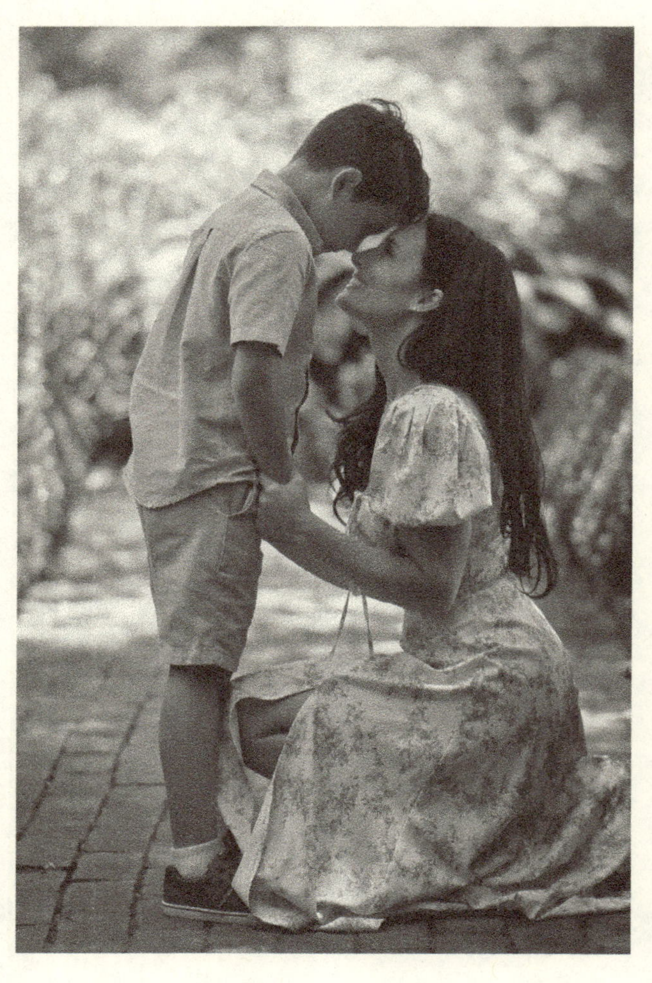

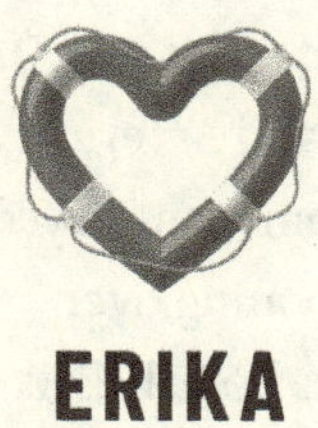

ERIKA

Erika was the first "official" ship mom I interviewed, in August 2017. I didn't tell her she was the first. I acted like I had done these interviews a thousand times. If I watch the tape of our first interview, I cringe at myself initially, but Erika, a consummate performer, was comfortable and chatty, which helped my nerves. Her story was sweet and romantic, and I always returned to it as a possibility for one of the book's selected stories. At the beginning of 2021, I connected with her again. After that interview—and learning what her family had gone through since our last chat—I knew her story needed to be in this book.

Erika—from Key West, Florida—joined ships as a singer after working two jobs and touring around California with her band. She wanted nothing more than to sing professionally, so when she stumbled across an ad looking for cruise-ship singers, she applied immediately. In the spring of 2010, she joined the Carnival crew and immediately loved it on board.

She got her own cabin and was grateful for the experience of working with such great musicians while travelling.

She kept thinking, *Is this my life?*

A few years into ship life, she met Daniel in Alaska, on board *Westerdam*, owned by Holland America. He was working on board but from the UK: a handsome, blue-eyed, bearded cadet that the female crew had been swooning over.

Days after arriving on board, Erika sat beside him in the theatre during a show. He tells everyone she was playing footsie with him during that show. She says she was just re-adjusting herself. Either way, the instant chemistry between them was undeniable. They spent the rest of the night chatting and getting to know one another. He talked about how he was getting the crew together to go out and clean the beaches the next day, after a recent tsunami had left them covered in garbage.

Erika was utterly exhausted—she had just joined *Westerdam*, immediately after leaving another ship—but when Daniel asked if she'd like to join him, she felt energized. She batted her eyelashes and said, "Yes, of course!"

The next day was a magical first date. They cleaned beaches on stunning islands in Alaska, with humpback whales jumping in the background. They shared their first kiss on the ship's stern. They fell for each other hard and quickly, and Erika found herself introducing Daniel to her mother, who came on board only a week later. A month later, she admitted she was in love with him.

Like many ship couples, they knew their time together had an expiry date. Daniel was set to go back home to the marine academy in the UK to finish up his cadetship, and Erika was set to go on board *Volendam* to travel Asia and Australia. As they sailed into the remarkable Fossil Point in Tuxedni Bay, also called "Alaska's Jurassic Park," both were completely distraught and unable to enjoy it, even with the *Jurassic Park* theme song playing in the background.

Apart, they spent months talking every day and travelling crazy distances to be together when they could. In the spring of 2013, he ended up flying to Japan to join her on board for a visit. It was then they decided they would be together and make it work no matter what—which in their case, because they were from different countries, included getting a marriage visa before he properly proposed. It wasn't the most romantic way to get engaged, so Daniel would randomly propose to Erika on walks or at the grocery store to try to make up for it. It obviously worked, because they were married on April 26, 2014. She walked down the aisle to the *Jurassic Park* theme song.

From then on, Erika and Daniel worked and travelled together on cruise ships. Daniel worked his way up to navigation officer, responsible for the navigational operations of the ship, and Erika continued to sing and perform. They were thrilled when Erika got pregnant while they were on a vacation in England and were so happy to start their family.

Once back on board, Erika worked until she was six months pregnant and then travelled to Budapest to sing in a friend's wedding as promised. She then made her way back to England with plans arranged to go home to Florida to have the baby and wait for Daniel to finish up his current contract on board. Unfortunate timing brought Hurricane Irma, a Category 5 hurricane that caused widespread destruction across its path.

Erika arrived back in Key West just in time for the city to be evacuated, forcing her to go to an aunt's home in West Palm Beach. There she had an allergic reaction to the family cat and had to get rushed to hospital. The drive there was harrowing, with the route surrounded by falling trees, pole lines, and other debris left from the storm.

Sadly, Irma completely wiped out the house that Erika had set up for the arrival of the baby. She ended up staying with friends in Pennsylvania while things got repaired in Key West. With Daniel finally off the ship, they eventually bought a trailer and renovated it when she was eight months pregnant. Their sweet boy, Ezra, was born a month later. The family ended up buying a house in North Carolina that they would live in when not travelling.

Ezra first came on board when he was six months old. He had a bunch of firsts on board—walking, swimming, a haircut, and his first birthday. The family loved being at sea and felt it was a great opportunity for their son to explore the world and other cultures. What better way to teach the history of the Roman Colosseum than to go there?

As for most families around the world, things took a big turn for Erika's family in 2020. Arrangements were underway for Ezra to start school on land while Erika got back to focusing on her singing and acting career. Daniel hooked a job on superyachts, changing his time at sea from three months on, three months off to two months on, two months off. The family planned to do one last run on board cruise ships before adjusting to their new life.

Though 2020 had been forecast to be a record year for cruising, with over thirty-two million passengers, that was all about to change.

Erika remembers Daniel's dad voicing concern when the situation unfolding in China seemed to be getting worse. "I don't think you guys should go on the ship right now," he said. Assuming, like we all did, that this pandemic was not going to spread worldwide, the family travelled to the Civitavecchia port near Rome, Italy, to join *Nieuw Statendam* in the spring of 2020.

For the first month, it was fine. But things started looking serious when a bunch of charter passengers scheduled to come on board started cancelling. After every charter had cancelled, there were no more passengers. Just the crew was left on board. Minus the entertainers because there were no passengers to entertain. At the beginning, no one was fazed. Everyone thought the pandemic would pass soon enough.

I've said that all crew members are well versed in protocols for illness. We follow an outbreak prevention plan, which is the guide for preventing and responding to any outbreak of illness on board. When a breakout occurs, everyone—no matter what their job or status—has to help. I admit that it was sometimes fun to watch stuck-up staff members serve food in the guest buffet, but it was a major pain to sanitize every surface for days on end.

On Daniel and Erika's ship, everyone was social distancing. But the pool was open, so it became an area where they could socialize, and Ezra learned to swim without his floaties. As the only kid on board with a thousand-plus crew members, he got a lot of attention. And more than a thousand willing babysitters. The ship wasn't equipped with enough face masks, though, so the crew in laundry started manufacturing reusable ones. Ezra had pint-size masks made for him, which Erika drew moustaches on.

On board, things quickly went from bad to worse as the number of COVID cases started increasing around the globe and countries started locking down. Cruise ships became the last thing any port wanted to see docking, and suddenly, only selected countries were allowing ships to disembark.[13] The US Centers for Disease Control and Prevention (CDC) started implementing new rules for the ships, requiring crew members to always stay in their cabins and shutting down all access to common areas, such as the pool and the gym.[14]

On Erika's ship, once it had been acknowledged that the crew were being asked to spend their time in their windowless cabins, unable to eat outside of them or to walk the promenade, it was decided that the crew would be moved up to the balcony guest cabins so they could have fresh air and daylight. Although that helped a lot, the crew grew nervous about the future of their jobs—and even more nervous about not knowing how long it would be before their feet could touch land. The cruise industry was falling apart, and the crew were stuck out at sea.

Luckily, Ezra was almost done potty training as Erika started to run low on items. Amazon orders had been cancelled because there was no way to get packages to the ship. That changed once the ship arrived in Fort Lauderdale. The port authority agents there went above and beyond. They not only got diapers, wipes, and supplies to Erika but also drove her car around the lot once a week to ensure that it didn't seize up. (Erika's family members had taken her car to the port and had given the keys to the port agents.)

Daniel was run off his feet working and had to start eating in a different area with the other essential ship operators, to socially distance themselves. This meant that Erika was on parenting duty almost all the time, which was challenging. However, Daniel took every opportunity to take Ezra on walks around the ship decks.

With their toddler, the couple coped as well as they could under the circumstances. Erika spent countless hours sitting in the cabin with Ezra, trying to kill the time with art, games, or movies. But even in her large passenger room, the walls were closing in. For her sanity and a space that was all her own, Erika started what she called *Melodies at Sea*. Every day, she would post a video of herself on her YouTube channel, singing a song in the cabin.[15] Bonus: it showed their family and friends that they were okay. Day one was March 29, 2020, when she gave a powerful performance of "Never Enough" from The Greatest Showman. Under the YouTube video, she wrote, "A daily dose of hopeful rhythms, keeping us connected."[16]

With everything so in limbo, at random times, information would rapidly spread through the ship. Some crew from specific countries were transferring to different ships that would get them on flights back to their countries. Maybe. Because Erika's family's ship had a healthy crew who were taking their temperatures and logging everything twice a day, it was frustrating that they couldn't just walk off the ship into their countries. Instead, they would have to board flights, putting themselves and everyone else at risk to get home.

When singing again was just starting to make Erika feel a little normal, the family got hit with the news that they would be split up. Erika and Ezra, along with the other American and Canadian crew, were set to disembark Daniel's ship onto a Princess Cruises ship containing all North Americans. Not only did they have to move to another ship, but also the transfer had to be done via a small cruise-ship tender boat in the middle of the Atlantic Ocean. Erika admitted that she cried a lot, but once the captain had explained that the ship was heading to Europe and things would become even more complicated for the crew there, she started packing their things and focusing on getting herself and her boy back on land.

As the navigational officer on board, Daniel drove the tender that took the North American crew over to their new-for-now boat. Ezra sat on his dad's lap while he drove, honking and waving goodbye to the *Nieuw Statendam*. When the tender hit the open ocean, the waves picked up, and it bobbed in the water. The turbulence started making everyone feel uneasy, and Ezra cried and gripped onto Daniel, who was concentrating hard on delivering them safely. When they finally arrived at the new ship, the family hugged, kissed, cried, and said goodbye.

When asked which day sticks out as a particularly hard day during the lockdown, Erika said that this was undoubtedly the one.

Luckily, her day did start to get better. Although Erika didn't know anyone on board the Princess ship, the hotel director was more than welcoming and had arranged an amazing suite for her and Ezra. As additional bonuses, they had free internet—gold to any crew member—and the captain's two children were also on board.

Erika told me that when she finally dropped her bags in that room, she could finally exhale and breathe again. She knew they were safe.

Everyone on board was a little uneasy and anxious, never knowing what was going to happen next. Plans were made and cancelled, and no one knew if they were coming or going. Erika's therapeutic *Melodies at Sea* continued on board the new ship, with the backdrop changing from a white couch to a navy-blue bed.

One day, when chatting with someone about their frustration that the US wouldn't let their healthy countrymen disembark, Erika sang about what they had been discussing to the tune of the chorus of "How Far I'll Go" in Disney's *Moana*: [17]

"We, the guests and the crew here on board, we're calling. We want to come home. Please let us come home . . . "

She went back to her cabin and wrote a parody of the song in twenty minutes. Then she recorded the video on her balcony, with the ocean behind her:

"I've been staring down at the water, long as I can remember.
Is today going to be the day?
I wish I could hear over the PA *that you're going home today.*
Everything is going to be okay.
Everyday at sea that we're not let in keeps me wondering why we're not let in
Even though we're clean and we're citizens.
It's just not okay . . .
We, the guests and the crew here on board, we're calling.
We want to come home. Please let us come home.
To the land of the free.
Hey, we're clean and we're healthy,
Just let us come home.

And my car's in port so I can just drive it home.
I know everybody there in office has a hand in this process,
Could you be the one to get us home?
Forty-five days at sea with a toddler is fun at times, but at others, obviously not ideal.
We all sanitize, wear our masks inside; social distance–wise, we should get a prize.
We all do our part. Have it in your heart. Let us come back home.
We, the guests and the crew here on board, we're calling.
We want to come home. Please let us come home.
To the land of the free.
Hey, we're clean and we're healthy,
Just let us come home.
We want to come home.
We're Americans and Canadians . . ."

The video ends with a quick shot of Erika and Ezra on the balcony, with the ocean in the background, as far as the eye can see.

Weeks later, just when Erika and the crew thought they might not be able to take it anymore, the announcement they had all been waiting for came over the PA. The captain told them that they would all be able to disembark in Fort Lauderdale. The ship erupted with applause and screams. It was finally going to be over.

On their fifty-sixth day on board the two ships, Erika posted her thirty-eighth and final Melodies at Sea video. She had saved her rendition of Andrea Bocelli's song "Time to Say Goodbye" for the special occasion.

The game plan was for Erika and Ezra to go to Key West and quarantine. When the duo finally disembarked, she felt a little scared leaving her healthy, constantly monitored ship bubble. Land life looked much different now. She was nervous entering the country with the highest COVID numbers in the world and too many people who thought it was all a hoax. Once again, the amazing workers at the port authority helped Erika by putting gas in her car and having it ready for her to leave right away for her four-hour trip. Erika and Ezra stayed in Key West for a month and then followed the travel plan to get back home to North Carolina.

Daniel surprised them two months later, banging on the front door of their home at midnight, startling his wife and son out of bed. Ezra jumped in his arms like no time had passed. Erika said when she laid eyes on her husband, it was like a dream.

When I caught up with Erika in 2024, she told me she is still performing: singing and acting. She was given five best-actress awards from different festivals around the world for her part in the 2023 short thriller *Overshadow*. She often travels to Colorado or LA for film shoots, and although she'll always be an active singer, she loves acting.

I learned that Erika's family has grown, with the addition of another sweet boy, named Luca. It was a planned pregnancy this time around, so it was a very different, much calmer pregnancy compared to her travelling pregnancy with Ezra. Erika continued singing with her band until she was eight months pregnant. She also sits on the board of a charter school that Ezra attends, which she helped to get up and running. Life is busy for their family, but it's wonderfully busy.

Daniel continues to work at sea but on private mega yachts, currently out of Germany. (She hinted at how his last employer was a celebrity but couldn't disclose the name. Of course, I wanted the dirt, but I didn't pry it out of her.) He still loves the work and will likely continue to work on ships until he retires. He currently does two months on and two months off, which is a great schedule for any seafarer.

The couple is apart a lot. However, the family members are used to their nomad life, which works well for them. They keep their love fresh by having regular date nights when together, and Erika admits that the frequent distance also keeps the couple's passion ablaze. While Luca is still too young to understand, Ezra does get sad when his dad leaves for work. But he takes it like a champ and knows that when Daniel is gone, he's the man of the house and sweetly helps his mom. Erika said that when Daniel is home, he's the most hands-on dad there is and that she and his children absolutely adore him.

The reality is that fathers like Daniel are the exception and not the rule when it comes to the stories of ship moms. Many ship kids never get to meet their biological fathers, and that's a shame. I wanted to make sure to celebrate the great fathers, like Daniel, who are making it work and being wonderful role models for their children. While this book commemorates mothers, the great fathers also deserve their flowers.

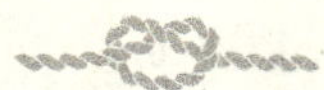

In writing Erika's story, I thought I would be doing crew members around the world a major disservice by not talking about what other seafarers experienced during the COVID-19 pandemic. Not everyone was as lucky as Erika's family, and she'd be the first to admit it. You get a lot of extra perks when you have the only kid on board.

When the pandemic started, the World Health Organization announced that "more than half of corona cases outside China" were on a single cruise ship, the *Diamond Princess*.[18] With about thirty-seven hundred people on board, more than seven hundred got infected and thirteen people died.[19] Thousands of people in close quarters make cruise ships ideal for potential infection spread. The world started looking at ships as "floating cesspools," and the CDC started locking the cruise-ship industry down.

In March 2020, the United States Coast Guard reported 80,000 souls stuck in 122 ships in US waters alone.[20] They would then try to disembark in ports, only to be vilified, rejected, and sent away when the ships were sitting close enough to jump onto land. Cruise lines that tried to repatriate their crew encountered CDC regulations and the government policies of different countries, making it almost impossible for some crew to make it home.[21]

There was no rhyme or reason to what happened from ship to ship or from cruise line to cruise line, and there were many different experiences. Some crew said it depended on your nationality. Some said it depended on how many stripes you had.

Like Erika, online, I saw crew move to passenger cabins with patios and post the most incredible photos of sunsets and ships from different fleets floating together and anchored outside unwelcoming ports. Some crew decided to stay on board willingly, as they felt more comfortable there than back home in their countries, riddled with COVID-19 and bad leadership.

I could see a lot of people struggling with mental health and was broken-hearted to see report after report of crew suicides. I saw photos of crew members protesting on a pool deck, holding up bed sheets spray-painted with, "How do you sleep at night?" and "How many more suicides do you need?"

I saw videos of crew crying and pleading in airports, stranded in countries that weren't their own—without proper visas, money, food, or accommodations. There were posts from crew isolated in tiny, prison-like cabins for weeks. With no windows, Wi-Fi, or cell service, the crew had difficulty determining whether it was day or night. Also keep in mind that all these stressed-out people were now receiving little to no salary. In some cases, people were unable to feed their families.

Enter people like Caitlin Vaughn, program manager with the International Seafarers' Welfare and Assistance Network (ISWAN). During the pandemic, on January 18, 2021, I spoke to her via Zoom. She was working from home, helping these seafarers. ISWAN is a non-profit organization that promotes the welfare and well-being of crew around the world with a number of projects and programs. Their primary service is their free, twenty-four-hour, multilingual helpline for seafarers and their families.

ISWAN reported that their helpline cases tripled during the COVID-19 pandemic.[22] All the staff are trained in providing emotional support, counselling, suicide risk assessments, and more. They also have two certified counsellors and a network of clinical psychologists. Staff are prepared with the most common crew languages, such as Filipino, Russian, Hindi, Chinese, Spanish, and Arabic, and translators of other languages are on hand if required. This support has been an invaluable resource for the crew, so much so that they have now expanded the service to accommodate superyacht crews with their dedicated helpline. Caitlin admitted that the ISWAN helpline staff—feeling helpless and frustrated—also struggled with their own mental health during that time.

Apart from helping seafarers with mental health, this organization also assisted seafarers with financial support. For example, Caitlin told me that 2,000 crew members who were stranded in dormitories in Manila during the lockdown received food supplies with the Seafarers' Emergency Fund. Altogether, some 330 Filipino seafarers and their families received US$500 through the ISWAN Hardship Fund. The organization even arranged special flights for stranded crew members to return to their home countries.

Sadly, the statistics on how many crew members decided to take their lives during the pandemic will remain unknown. No marine administration enforces the reporting of deaths at sea. During our conversation, Caitlin advised me that ISWAN is lobbying to change that by asking the International Labour Organization for a central reporting system.

With confirmed reports of an increase in the numbers of people calling hotlines with suicidal thoughts—and every few days, seeing a new obituary on ship-crew Facebook pages—I feel frustrated to have no number to report. Class-action lawsuits have been filed against some cruise lines for failure to protect their crew members (and passengers) during the lockdown.[23]

If you or someone you know is a struggling crew member, SeafarerHelp is available twenty-four hours a day, 365 days a year. Direct-dial +44 20 7323 2737, chat online at www.seafarerhelp.org, or email help@seafarerhelp.org.[24]

Please. Do it.

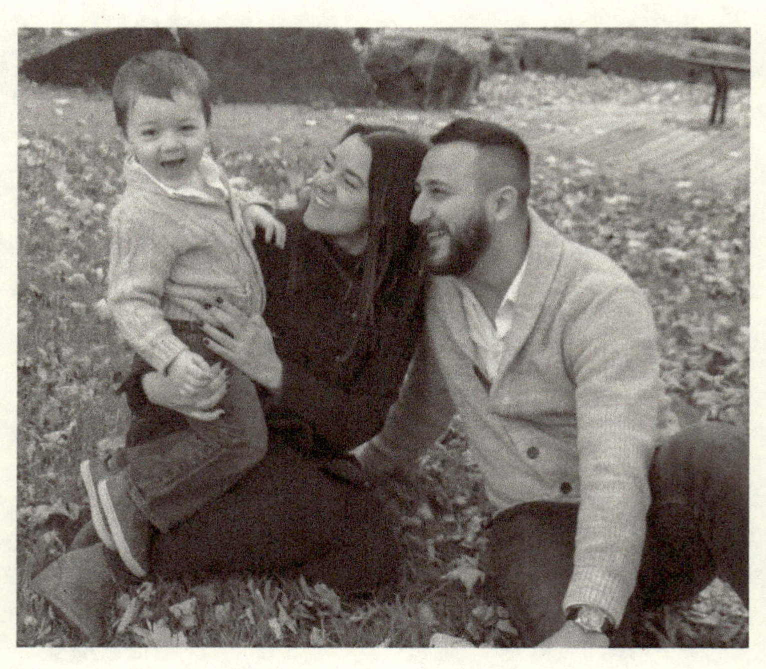

Even more today than when I was on board, I look at each cruise ship, once just a vessel, as a beating heart of dedicated individuals who breathe life into its every corner. The true essence of life working on cruise ships lies not just in the destinations but in the stories and bonds forged along the way. Those on board who continue to work tirelessly behind the scenes, ensuring that the magic on the surface remains seamless and enchanting, deserve recognition for their hard work and dedication.

As I type the final pages of this journey through the world of ship moms, a surge of emotions goes through me. What began as an idea to connect with others transformed into a collection of tales that I'm honoured to have been entrusted with. Your background doesn't matter. Across cultures, everybody just wants to belong, to be respected, to love and be loved. The journey has been a humbling and transformative experience.

There were so many beautiful stories that it's possible other books may stem from this project. Time will tell. I would love to interview more ship moms, airline crew, and more.

This book would not have been possible without all the ship moms who shared with me—the ship moms featured in the individual chapters of this book. They each gave me something specific to reflect upon. Erika, Janete, Dani, Melodie, Tanya, Sage, Lee-Ann, Margarita, and Arlene were not paid a cent to chat with me, some of them for many hours. Although I had no money to offer, they all agreed to share with me. Without them, this whole project would not be possible.

I hope they know how much gratitude I have—and how much respect. I will always sing their praises for being some of the most incredible women I have ever had the privilege of getting to know. If this book does really well, rest assured, reader. These moms will also reap the financial benefits. (Although even the most "successful" books are often not financially successful for the authors, a girl can dream.) Unless this thing becomes the next *Eat Pray Love*, I know that my bank account will likely remain scanty.

I even dream of starting a ship-moms foundation, to which underprivileged pregnant crew members can apply and receive some financial assistance. That, of course, is thinking big. But this book was just a dream at one point, and here we are. Anything is possible.

Life moves quickly. Gabriel is now seven years old and growing like a weed. He calls me "*Mamãe*," Portuguese for "Mommy," and I love that. Every night, we sing him to sleep in both languages. He is losing his babyish ways and, sadly, no longer calls jeans "jeams" and gloves "glubs," and it breaks my heart. But he has started calling his vitamins "vitamints," so there's hope he'll remain my little boy a while longer.

Being a mom is the best, most challenging, most wonderful, most maddening thing ever. My little ADHD boy has tested me in every way, but I wouldn't change a thing. I've been surprised to find that, in some ways, I'm not as assured as I thought but that in others, I'm so much stronger than I ever knew I could be. Being a mom has helped me learn more about myself than anything else I've ever done.

My former husband has re-married and now has a daughter of his own. In the October 2015 journal entry that opened this book, I wrote that I would someday "see him online with his beautiful family. I hope I feel joy for him and not regret."

I do feel joy for him.

Like my ex, his wife and child are thin, blond, beautiful, and very happy. Luiz, Gabriel, and I are all dark-haired with curves, and our opposite-looking families have been more than cordial when seeing each other at mutual friends' weddings. When I was in my previous relationship, I didn't think there was such a thing as coming back from cheating, and I was the culprit. Now, even with the tables turned, I can say that some couples can come back from it—if they want it enough.

To everyone's shock—including mine—Luiz and I are still together and in love. While I continue to work in non-profit arts, he works in non-profit immigration, offering settlement and integration services to immigrants and refugees. We both love and feel fulfilled by our jobs, but we continue to struggle with money. He misses Brazil, his family, and his friends, and his father has recently had some health issues. I tell him I would move to Brazil in a heartbeat, but he says he wants to stay here for Gabriel.

We had not been to Brazil in six years. The pandemic hasn't helped. However, we have diligently saved our money, and the three of us escaped the Canadian cold, making our way to Rio de Janeiro for a month in spring 2025. Gabriel, who loves nothing more than talking, did a good job under the circumstances, not being able to speak to his friends and his Brazilian family members. He did pick up a lot of Portuguese while there, namely "*vem cá, Vovó*" ("come here, Grandma") and every popular swear word and curse phrase.

During the trip, I was in the final stages of preparing this book for publication, so Gabriel spent time with his grandmother, and with his grandfather Luiz and his new wife, Sandra—as well as his great-grandmother and numerous other wonderful and welcoming family members. As Gabriel wasn't even two years old the first time we met everyone, my heart burst thinking about all the memories he made during our stay. We're already discussing the next trip and have promised to try to make it back in a couple of years.

Luiz's parents and family constantly communicate with and adore their rambunctious Canadian boy. I continue to feel a strong connection, particularly to Luiz's mom, Paula, who exudes love and support from Petrópolis to us daily. I hope to spend more time with her to learn from her, namely how to sew and cook. Of course we have a language barrier, but we make it work. She's currently taking English lessons, and I'm aiming to be more fluent by the next trip.

Recently, while Luiz was wearing headphones while doing dishes, he was on the phone, chatting with his mom. Feeling silly, thinking he was listening to his podcasts and not noticing he was on the phone, I came up in front of him and flashed him my boobs, in full display of the phone camera. It wasn't a quick flash but rather a little dance with my shirt up over my head, bare boobs flopping freely. When I finally looked at Luiz, he was wide-eyed with a Cheshire grin. He slightly glanced toward the phone screen. This was when I saw Paula covering her eyes and mouth in obvious fits of laughter. As we say in Newfoundland, "I handy died."

It took a week or so before I could even look at her again, and when I did, it was because she made me. She told me she loved to see that we were so playful together, in love and having fun. She also told me I had nice boobs.

In a solid relationship, you should look for consistency, authenticity, accountability, sincerity, respect, passion, humour—and, of course, love. Tall order? Yes.

We're two people from very different backgrounds and whose ages shouldn't match. Yet we have matched perfectly and even lived through a pandemic to tell the tale. That's why I feel so lucky. Of course, Luiz and I still drive each other crazy sometimes, but I never doubt him and our relationship. Once unsure of myself, I'm now so confident in our partnership that I never worry about or second-guess anything.

I am completely myself and no longer even think about the age difference—unless I'm patting myself on the back for bagging such a young hottie.

NOTES

[1] https://www.lipcon.com/blog/rising-crimes-on-cruise-ships/

[2] https://www.womenonwaves.org/en/page/938/vessel--documentary-about-wow

[3] https://www.politico.com/newsletters/politico-nightly/2024/04/08/deconstructing-trumps-abortion-statement-00151147
https://www.facebook.com/thedailyshow/videos/trump-attacks-dems-on-abortion/3280823585557289/

[4] https://www.bbc.com/news/world-latin-america-52719391

[5] https://www.bbc.com/news/world-latin-america-52080830

[6] https://www.usmagazine.com/entertainment/pictures/below-deck-sailings-jean-luc-wants-to-coparent-with-dani/

[7] https://www.usmagazine.com/celebrity-moms/news/below-decks-dani-soares-opens-up-about-motherhood-mental-health/

[8] https://people.com/parents/below-deck-jean-luc-cerza-lanaux-dani-soares-address-baby-news/#:~:text=%22I%20want%20everybody%20to%20know,do%20with%20that%20child's%20life

[9] https://www.instagram.com/p/CPc-7J1r7_u/?utm_source=ig_embed&ig_rid=53264d61-128b-4b40-a18d-8c0712150b08

[10] https://www.usmagazine.com/celebrity-moms/news/below-decks-jean-luc-cerza-lanaux-breaks-silence-over-danis-baby/

[11] https://www.usmagazine.com/celebrity-news/news/kate-chastain-shades-jean-luc-amid-dani-soares-baby-daddy-rumors/

[12] https://people.com/parents/below-deck-sailing-yacht-jean-luc-cerza-lanaux-confirms-father-dani-soares-baby/

[13] https://southpacificislands.travel/coronavirus-which-cruise-ports-are-closed/

[14] https://www.miamiherald.com/news/business/tourism-cruises/article242565281.html

[15] https://www.youtube.com/watch?v=94YBbrbqa8A&list=PLCYtg7fPbphmRHqXXsBdHXkfj6_E_VyfB&index=38

[16] https://www.youtube.com/watch?v=94YBbrbqa8A&list=PLCYtg7fPbphmRHqXXsBdHXkfj6_E_VyfB&index=39

[17] https://qz.com/1852646/tens-of-thousands-are-still-stuck-on-cruise-ships

[18] https://www.theguardian.com/world/live/2020/feb/20/coronavirus-live-updates-diamond-princess-cruise-ship-japan-deaths-latest-news-china-infections

[19] https://english.kyodonews.net/news/2025/02/044a4a592087-former-diamond-princess-passengers-mark-5-yrs-since-covid-outbreak.html#google_vignette

[20] https://www.cbc.ca/news/business/cruise-ships-stranded-crew-members-cdc-covid-19-1.5552424

[21] https://www.cbc.ca/news/business/cruise-ships-stranded-crew-members-cdc-covid-19-1.5552424

[22] https://www.iswan.org.uk/news/helpline-cases-triple-as-seafarers-seek-help-during-covid-19-pandemic/

[23] https://www.expertinstitute.com/resources/insights/cruise-lines-face-lawsuits-from-passengers-and-crew-over-covid-19-outbreaks/

[24] https://www.iswan.org.uk/seafarerhelp/

ACKNOWLEDGEMENTS

First, I want to sincerely thank the two loves of my life—Luiz Dutra and our boy, Gabriel—for their encouragement and support during this challenging process. You make me so happy.

I am so grateful to my family for their unwavering support: my sisters, Lisa Winsor and Sam Winsor; my parents, Al Winsor and Verna Hart; my brother, Craig Bulger; and my niece and nephew, Emily and Liam. Thanks to my wonderful, large Brazilian family—with special thanks to Paula Dutra and Luiz Cláudio. I love you all so much. *Te amo*!

My heartfelt thanks to Rebecca Rose and the team at Breakwater Books, my number-one choice, for taking a chance on me. I hope to make you proud and sell some books. To my substantive editor Leslie Vryenhoek, I can't thank you enough for helping me shake off my nerves with your insightful edits. Thank you for believing in my story and enhancing it in ways I never imagined! Big thanks to my copy editor Shelley Egan for her eagle eye. I'm so grateful for your support and expertise!

Thanks to the two sweethearts in my trifecta, Virginia Fudge and Allison Graham, without whom this book would not have happened. Allison, you got me onto cruise ships and gave me the idea to write this book. Virginia, you've been a significant source of strength from the beginning of this project, giving me motivation and an invaluable artistic perspective.

Thanks to Kelley Power and Amanda Labonté for your warm welcome into the literary industry, with support, encouragement, and laughs. Big thanks to my girl Wendy Rose. Your support with social media and promotions was beyond helpful. Thanks to Andrea Hyde, pea in my pod and super librarian friend, for strengthening my work with your notes and keeping our book club going after all these years. Thanks to Ray Critch for your assistance and skills! I am honoured to be a Breakwater author with you! Thanks to Don-E Coady, for always inspiring and pushing me to work harder. Thank you to my WritersNL colleagues, organizational committees, and boards for the hard work and moral support over the years. Thanks to the authors who chatted with me about the project and gave me advice, including Ainsley Hawthorn, Edward Riche, Andrew Peacock, Kerri Cull, Joel Thomas Hynes, Susie Taylor, Terry Doyle, Carolyn Parsons, and many more.

Thanks to Erin Martin, who, unbeknownst to her, has been a driving force, encouraging me to embrace my over-the-top dreams. Erin, I haven't seen you in twenty years, but once, smoking outside the Goulds Rec Centre, you told me that I was going to do great things. You said it so matter-of-factly, so confidently, that I believed it. Sometimes, when my inner saboteur tries to stop me from taking big steps, I think, *Screw you, saboteur! Erin*

Martin thinks I'm special, so I'm doing this, dammit! This book is a huge example of one of those things. So thank you, Erin, for proof that kind words can go a long way.

Thanks to my music industry mentor—the late, great icon Denis Parker—with whom I shared book recommendations and who always supported me. I wish that I could have read your book and that you could have read this one.

Thanks to all the ship crew across all cruise lines who work hard every day for the guests. I hope you enjoy these stories from your colleagues! Thanks to my many ship friends around the world. Thanks to Josip from the Crew Center for spreading the word to the ship moms and to Ross Klein from Cruise Junkie for your guidance and expertise. Big thanks to Amber Eaton and the *Serenade of the Seas* for the fantastic backdrop of the ship in my hometown for the book's photoshoot. And thanks to Ritche Perez for your superb photography skills on board.

Thanks to my Fogo family for letting me use Nan and Pop's house for my writing retreat. Nan and Pop Combden, I hope you're watching down on me and are proud of my hard work. And I hope you aren't mad at me for smoking pot on your stoop.

Lastly, my deepest gratitude to all the ship moms around the world who shared their stories with me. Special thanks to the ladies who have appeared in this book and to those who are featured: Erika, Janete, Dani, Melodie, Lee-Ann, Arlene, Margarita, Tanya, and Sage. I cannot thank you all enough for your time and willingness to open up to me.

The land on which *Ship Moms* was completed, Newfoundland and Labrador, is the ancestral homeland of the Beothuk, Mi'kmaq, Innu of Nitassinan, Inuit of Nunatsiavut, and Inuit of

NunatuKavut. It is important to me to acknowledge the diverse Indigenous Peoples who continue to live in this province and to recognize them as past, present, and future caretakers.

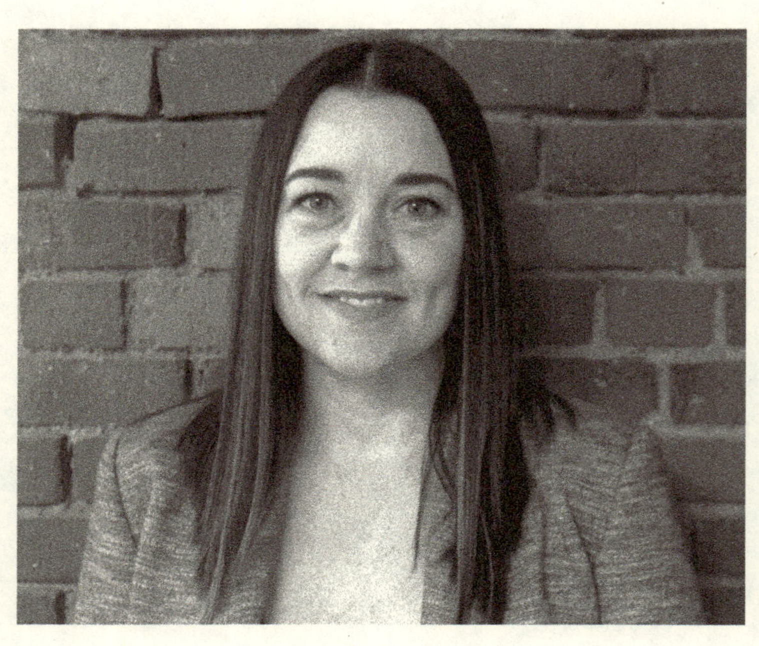

THE AUTHOR

Jen Winsor is an arts administrator who has worked in the Newfoundland and Labrador arts scene for almost twenty years, focusing on music and literature. Jen left the province to travel with Royal Caribbean Cruise Lines Arts and Entertainment Division, but her plans were cut short when she got pregnant, with a crew member twelve years younger than her. Returning to her home province, she happily became the executive director of WritersNL. When she's not lost in a book or typing up funding applications, you'll find her hiking the East Coast Trail, enjoying a drag show, or experiencing some live music. Jen lives in St. John's with her son, Gabriel, and his ridiculously good-looking Brazilian dad, Luiz.